The Diabetic Gourmet Cookbook

More Than 200 Healthy Recipes from Homestyle Favorites to Restaurant Classics

Editors of
Diabetic Gourmet Magazine

WILEY
John Wiley & Sons, Inc.

Published by John Wiley & Sons, Inc., Hoboken, New Jersey
Published simultaneously in Canada

Design and production by Navta Associates Inc.

Diabetic Gourmet is a registered trademark of CAPCO Marketing.

For general information about our other products and services, please contact our Customer Care Department within the United States at (800) 762-2974, outside the United States at (317) 572-3993 or fax (317) 572-4002.

Wiley also publishes its books in a variety of electronic formats. Some content that appears in print may not be available in electronic books. For more information about Wiley products, visit our web site at www.wiley.com.

Library of Congress Cataloging-in-Publication Data

The diabetic gourmet cookbook : more than 200 healthy recipes from homestyle favorites to restaurant classics / editors of the Diabetic Gourmet Magazine.
    p. cm.
  Includes bibliographical references and index.
  ISBN 0-471-39326-6 (paper)
  1. Diabetes—Diet therapy—Recipes. 2. Diabetes—Diet therapy. I. Diabetic Gourmet Magazine.
  RC662.D537 2004
  641.5'6314—dc22

                      2004003681

Printed in the United States of America
10 9 8 7 6 5 4 3 2 1

*To our families, cherished readers, and the
millions of people living with diabetes*

Contents

Preface

First of all, don't let the title of this book scare you. While *The Diabetic Gourmet Cookbook* has been designed to meet the needs of people living with diabetes, it really is a cookbook for everyone who appreciates great food. With over 200 recipes that are perfect for everyday meals, as well as for entertaining, *The Diabetic Gourmet Cookbook* makes a wonderful, thoughtful addition to any cookbook collection.

The recipes we have prepared are carefully portioned original creations, as well as modified versions of traditional favorites. They were created with a close eye on fat, calories, sodium, carbohydrate, and—last but definitely not least—taste. Complete with detailed nutritional information that includes diabetic food exchanges, the recipes allow readers to effectively and safely adhere to their meal plans or diets while enjoying delicious food. Even if you don't have diabetes or special dietary needs, you'll be able to feel good knowing that the food you're eating or serving to your family is as healthful as it is delicious.

Here at *Diabetic Gourmet Magazine,* we have long operated with the belief that the diabetic diet should be seen as selective, not restrictive. We also understand that while it is necessary for people living with diabetes to regulate their eating habits, it is unrealistic to expect them to suddenly not have a taste for certain types of food. By including healthier versions of the types of dishes that some would say helped them down the road to developing diabetes in the first place, *The Diabetic Gourmet Cookbook* addresses realistic food preferences in addition to healthy eating guidelines. After all, how many other health-oriented cookbooks have recipes for onion rings, pot roast, and baklava?

In *The Diabetic Gourmet Cookbook* we intend to focus on recipes while providing only the most basic information about diabetes, health, and meal planning. There are plenty of fantastic books and resources dedicated to diabetes and nutrition that provide in-depth, practical, and clinical information. We strongly advise anyone living with diabetes to buy a comprehensive book about the disease, preferably one that is endorsed by the American Diabetes Association.

The recipes provided in this cookbook were analyzed by Christine Capece using Professional Computer Planned Menus. When necessary, additional data was added using actual food labels from products and the USDA National Nutrient Database for Standard Reference.

Unless noted otherwise in a specific recipe, analysis was determined as follows:

- The larger number of servings was used when a range of servings was given.
- Suggested accompaniments are not included in analysis.
- When more than one ingredient is offered, such as "1 teaspoon nonfat mayonnaise, or 1 teaspoon light mayonnaise," the first ingredient was used for analysis.
- Optional ingredients were not included in analysis.
- Cooking sprays are either olive oil or canola oil based.
- Meat and poultry are considered fat-trimmed prior to cooking.

For those of you who still haven't seen *Diabetic Gourmet Magazine,* visit our Web site at DiabeticGourmet.com to find out what you've been missing. There are millions of other readers waiting to greet you!

Finally, I would like to thank our valued readers, our compadres, our partners in diabetes culinaria over the past several years for helping us do the things we love to do most. I hope you enjoy what we have prepared for you as much as we enjoyed preparing it.

Kirk N. Capece
Editor-in-chief,
Diabetic Gourmet Magazine

1

Diabetes Basics

Diabetes is a disease that makes it next to impossible for a person's body to convert the sugar it receives from food into energy. Normally, insulin is produced in the pancreas, and this insulin is needed to get the sugar into the cells for use as fuel. For a person living with diabetes, either the body doesn't produce enough insulin, or the body is unable to use the insulin that is produced. Without usable insulin, the body cannot get the energy it needs to function. This is what diabetes is all about—the inability of a person's body to get the energy it needs from food.

Signs and Symptoms

Millions of people have type 2 diabetes and don't even know it. By the time they are diagnosed, they have already lived with it for years, undiagnosed and untreated. How can this be? Many people exhibit no signs or symptoms of diabetes, and some of the symptoms they may have are mild enough to go unnoticed. Other times, people notice the symptoms, but they do not seem serious enough to cause them to contact a physician. In these cases, diabetes goes untreated for years, or until they visit a doctor for an ailment that developed as a result of their diabetes, such as blurred vision or numb fingers.

Early detection of diabetes is important because it can help prevent complications and damage to the body. According to the National Institute of Diabetes and Digestive & Kidney Diseases (NIDDK), all adults forty-five years old or older should get tested for diabetes, regardless of whether they have noticed any symptoms. People younger than forty-five should get tested if they display symptoms or if they have any of the high-risk characteristics that make them more prone to developing the disease.

In recent years, you may have heard the term "pre-diabetes." Pre-diabetes is used to classify people who are at a severe risk for developing type 2 diabetes. Fortunately, by making lifestyle changes such as eating healthier, adding moderate exercise or physical activity to their daily lives, and losing excess weight, people considered to be pre-diabetic can slow down or even prevent the onset of type 2 diabetes.

If you or a family member are experiencing the following symptoms, then you should consult a physician and get tested for diabetes as soon as possible.

- Increased or extreme hunger
- Increased urination
- Increased or excessive thirst
- Constant fatigue
- Changes in vision, such as blurred vision
- Unexpected weight loss
- Tingling or numbness in hands, fingers, or feet
- Cuts and sores that do not heal as quickly as they used to
- Higher incidence of infections

Types of Diabetes

There are two major types of diabetes, type 2 and type 1, as well as a third type called gestational diabetes, which occurs during a small percentage of pregnancies.

Type 2 diabetes is the most common form of diabetes, accounting for up to 95 percent of all cases. Formerly known as non–insulin-dependent diabetes mellitus (NIDDM) and as adult-onset diabetes, type 2 diabetes appears most often in middle-aged adults. However, there has been a disturbing trend in which young adults and adolescents are now developing it.

People develop type 2 diabetes because their pancreas either stops producing enough insulin to function, or because their body is no longer able to use the insulin it is producing (known as insulin resistance). Who is most at risk of developing type 2 diabetes?

- People who are overweight or obese
- People forty-five years old or older

- People with a family history of diabetes
- People who are African American, Hispanic American, Native American, Asian American, or Pacific Islanders
- People who get little or no physical activity or exercise
- People with low HDL levels and high LDL levels
- Women who have delivered a baby weighing over nine pounds at birth

Type 1 diabetes accounts for about 5 percent of all cases of diabetes. Also commonly referred to as juvenile diabetes, or insulin-dependent diabetes mellitus (IDDM), it typically begins early in life with children and young adults suffering from an insulin deficiency.

The immune system of people with type 1 diabetes destroys the insulin-producing beta cells that are normally found in the pancreas. Because of this, people living with type 1 diabetes produce little or no insulin. They are therefore required to take insulin injections every day to replace the insulin their body is lacking.

The risk factors for developing type 1 diabetes are not as easily defined as those for type 2 diabetes, but they may include genetic and environmental factors.

Gestational diabetes develops in up to 5 percent of all pregnancies, but it usually goes away once the pregnancy has ended. However, women who develop gestational diabetes are at a higher risk of developing type 2 diabetes as they get older.

While the exact reason for developing gestational diabetes is not known, it is most common in women who have a family history of diabetes, who are obese when they get pregnant, or who are from a more diabetes-prone ethnic group. Hormones and hormonal changes at about the twenty-fourth week of pregnancy cause insulin resistance and can also lead to gestational diabetes. Women with gestational diabetes must take special precautions during pregnancy and work closely with their physicians to ensure a safe pregnancy.

Complications from Diabetes

People living with diabetes are at an increased risk for developing other health conditions or complications. The most common complications include heart disease, infections, nerve damage (neuropathy), kidney disease (nephropathy), and eye disease (retinopathy).

If you are a person with diabetes, any time you experience unexplained problems, such as headaches, blurred vision, or some of the symptoms mentioned earlier in this chapter, you should contact your doctor as soon as possible. It is important to stay in tune with your body and to be aware of possible warning signs alerting you about untreated health problems.

The best way to reduce the risk of complications is by controlling blood glucose levels. You can also reduce complications by eliminating high-risk behaviors that can lead to poor health. Add physical activity to your daily routine, quit smoking, lose excess weight, reduce your alcohol consumption, and eat healthier by cutting down on foods high in cholesterol, calories, and fat.

If you have already developed complications or have other health problems, then it is important that you closely follow the advice of your physician to help delay or prevent conditions from developing or worsening.

Treating Diabetes

The overall goal of diabetes treatment is to keep blood glucose levels as close to normal as possible. Keeping blood glucose levels under control reduces the risk of developing the life-threatening complications mentioned earlier, which is why it is so important to consistently test and monitor blood glucose levels.

When people with diabetes test their blood, they are actually testing to see how much sugar (glucose) has built up in their blood. When insulin is either ineffective or not being produced at all, glucose builds up in the blood and passes out of the body in the urine without being used. Even though the blood is loaded with glucose, the glucose doesn't make it into the cells and the body ends up losing its main source of energy. Testing blood sugar levels may not be pleasant and it may not always be convenient, but it is a very effective way to see how the body is reacting to the food people eat, the lifestyle they live, and the medications or treatments they have been prescribed.

Treatment of type 2 diabetes involves blood glucose level testing, a personalized meal plan, or diet and exercise. Prescribed oral medications or insulin may also be used to help control blood glucose levels.

Treatment of type 1 diabetes involves multiple daily injections of insulin, which are balanced with meals and daily activities. It includes frequent blood glucose level testing and a carefully designed and scheduled diet.

Managing Your Diabetes

It is important to remember that diabetes management needs to be addressed on an individual basis and that what may be good for one person with diabetes may not be good for another. Educating yourself on how to manage your diabetes is the best way to stay healthy. By sticking to a healthy diet, engaging in physical activity, and keeping a close eye on your health through frequent self-examination and regularly scheduled professional health examinations, you can effectively manage your diabetes and minimize complications.

To best manage your diabetes, you should organize a team of health care professionals so they can help you develop a personal diabetes-management plan that addresses personal issues such as lifestyle, diet, existing or developing health conditions, and medical care. Putting together a comprehensive, qualified team that you feel comfortable with may seem like a lot of work to go through, but it is definitely worth it. By providing you with information, resources, and coordinated treatment, your health care team can work together to help you manage your diabetes effectively.

In addition to your personal physician, a well-rounded health care team may include the following specialized professionals:

- Certified Diabetes Educator (C.D.E.)
- Certified Fitness Specialist
- Certified Wound Specialist
- Dermatologist
- Dietitian
- Neurologist
- Opthamologist
- Optometrist
- Pharmacist
- Podiatrist
- Psychologist or psychiatrist

We suggest that you begin by personally meeting with a Certified Diabetes Educator. A C.D.E. can help you get started and should be able to personally recommend other qualified professionals in your area.

For a more detailed look at the professionals whom you should include on your team, including additional resources relating to each specific profession, take a look at the Health Care Professionals section in the back of the book.

2

The Diabetic Pantry and Kitchen

Having a wide assortment of ingredients on your shelves will help you make more exciting meals and make meal planning easier. It will also help you get the variety of foods you need for a nutritious, well-balanced diet. Equipping yourself with the proper tools will make it more convenient to prepare your food using techniques that reduce fat and calories, as mentioned in chapter 3, Healthy Cooking Techniques. With the right collection of ingredients and tools, almost anyone can be a culinary success.

Individual preferences will ultimately dictate what your kitchen pantry contains. Your ethnic background and heritage, regional location, financial situation, and evolving cooking skills all shape your kitchen and your staple ingredients. Still, there are a number of ingredients and tools that we feel are both useful and essential in the kitchen and helpful to have when using this cookbook. We're including our suggestions here for you to consider.

Foods and Beverages

This section contains an extensive list of food items categorized according to the Diabetes Food Pyramid, as presented by the American Diabetes Association. For brief descriptions of these groupings, take a look at chapter 4, Meal Planning. With the exception of herbs, spices, and seasonings and certain condiments, which we have listed separately, each food group listed here contains items broken down into the following subcategories:

Pantry items. This subcategory includes dry and canned foods and other shelf-stable food items. This also includes fresh fruits and vegetables that generally do not require refrigeration. Many of these items will eventually become "refrigerator" items once they have been opened, but we'll be going by their status when bought. Examples include canned beans, couscous, and applesauce.

Refrigerator items. This subcategory includes items that are refrigerated when purchased and that have a shorter shelf life. Examples include milk and yogurt. We also include fresh vegetables that are generally refrigerated.

Freezer items. This subcategory includes three types of items: items that are frozen when purchased; items that are refrigerated when purchased, but that we recommend freezing so you have them on hand; and items that you prepare and then store in the freezer. Examples include fish fillets and homemade chicken broth.

This is by no means a definitive list of ingredients, and the appearance of an item below does not mean you can eat as much of it as you want. The items on this list offer variety and recommendations for certain products over others. The actual number of servings listed for each food grouping may not apply to everyone and every meal plan, so make sure you consult your dietitian for dietary recommendations suitable for you.

Vegetable Group (3 to 5 servings daily)

Pantry Items

Bamboo shoots, canned
Bean sprouts, canned
Ginger, sliced, pickled
Mushrooms, button, canned
Mushrooms, porcini, dried
Mushrooms, shitake, dried
Mushrooms, straw, canned
Onions, red
Onions, yellow or Vidalia
Peppers, jalapeño pepper rings, jar
Peppers, pepperoncini, jar
Peppers, roasted red peppers, jar
Potatoes, baking

Potatoes, new or red
Sauce, prepared tomato sauce, reduced or low-sodium
Shallots
Squash, yellow or green
Sweet potatoes or yams
Tomato paste, 8-ounce canned
Tomatoes, diced, reduced-sodium, canned
Tomatoes, fresh grape or cherry
Tomatoes, fresh Roma, plum or other
Tomatoes, puree, reduced-sodium, canned

Tomatoes, sun-dried, fresh, no oil added

Tomatoes, whole peeled Italian-style, reduced-sodium, canned

Tomatoes, whole peeled, reduced-sodium, canned

Water chestnuts, canned

Refrigerator Items

Carrots
Celery
Collard greens, fresh
Cucumber
Garlic, fresh bulbs

Ginger, fresh
Lettuce, green, red leaf, iceberg, or mesclun mix
Scallions
Spinach, fresh

Freezer Items

Artichoke hearts, 10-ounce package
Broccoli, chopped, 10-ounce package
Broth, vegetable, homemade, frozen in 1-cup to 2-quart containers

Marinara sauce, homemade
Spinach, chopped, 10-ounce package
Spinach, whole leaf, 10-ounce package
Peas, baby, 10-ounce package

Fruit Group (2 to 4 servings daily)

Pantry Items

Applesauce, unsweetened
Apples, fresh
Bananas, fresh
Cherries, dried
Cranberries, dried
Currants, dried
Dates, dried
Lemons, fresh
Limes, fresh
Oranges, fresh

Peaches, canned in juice (not syrup)
Pineapple chunks, canned in juice (not syrup)
Pineapple slices, canned in juice (not syrup)
Raisins, dark seedless
Raisins, golden seedless
Spreadable Fruit Spread, no-sugar added, various flavors

Refrigerator Items

Juice, 100% fruit juice such as orange and apple

Juice, lemon
Juice, lime

Freezer Items

Apple juice concentrate

Blueberries, unsweetened

Orange juice concentrate

Peaches, unsweetened

Raspberries or blackberries, unsweetened

Strawberries, unsweetened

Grains, Beans, and Starchy Vegetables (6 to 11 servings daily)

Pantry Items

Bagels, whole wheat preferred

Barley

Beans, black, low-sodium, canned

Beans, cannelloni, low-sodium, canned

Beans, garbanzo (chickpeas), low-sodium, canned or dry

Beans, kidney, white and red, low-sodium, canned or dry

Beans, navy, low-sodium, canned or dry

Beans, pinto, low-sodium, canned or dry

Bread crumbs, unseasoned

Breads, whole grain, various types including rye, whole wheat, and oat bran

Bulgur wheat

Cereals, high-fiber, low-sugar cereals such as bran flakes

Corn, baby, canned

Corn, kernels, low-sodium, canned

Oatmeal, various types including Scottish, Irish, and instant

Pasta, regular, various styles including penne and angel hair

Pasta, whole wheat, various styles including penne and rigatoni

Pasta, couscous

Pasta, orzo

Pasta, soba (long spaghetti style)

Pita bread, regular or whole wheat

Rice, basmati

Rice, brown, regular or quick-cooking

Rice, white, medium-grain, regular or quick-cooking

Squash, assorted winter varieties

Refrigerator Items

Biscuits, low-fat buttermilk

Freezer Items

Corn, kernels

Dough, phyllo

Milk Group (2 to 3 servings daily)

Pantry Items
Milk, nonfat, evaporated

Milk, nonfat, powdered

Refrigerator Items
Milk, nonfat
Sour cream, nonfat or light

Yogurt, fruit
Yogurt, plain low-fat

Freezer Items
Yogurt, frozen, nonfat

Meat and Other Group (2 to 3 servings daily)

Pantry Items
Almonds, sliced
Anchovies, canned
Cashews, whole unsalted
Clams, whole baby, canned
Peanuts, unsalted
Pecans, whole or sliced,
  unsalted

Pistachios, unsalted
Salmon, canned
Tuna, solid white albacore or
  chunk light, packed in water,
  canned
Walnuts, whole

Refrigerator Items
Cheese, hard cheeses such as
  Romano cheese
Cheese, nonfat or reduced-fat
  cream or Neufchâtel
Cheese, reduced-fat or part-
  skim mozzarella, Swiss, or
  Cheddar

Cheese, ricotta, part-skim or
  fat-free
Tofu, firm, reduced fat or lite
Turkey, deli-style, low-fat,
  low-sodium
Ham, deli-style, 97% fat-free

Freezer Items
Beef, ground, 95% to 97% lean
Broth, beef, homemade, frozen
  in 1-cup to 2-quart containers
Broth, chicken, homemade,
  frozen in 1-cup to 2-quart
  containers
Catfish, fillet (frozen in 3-ounce
  portions)

Chicken, boneless, skinless
  breast (pack 1 or 2 servings
  in a resealable plastic bag)
Chicken, cooked, cubed
Chicken, split breast, bone-in
Pork, bacon, reduced-fat,
  reduced-sodium
Pork, loin

Salmon, fillet (frozen in
    3-ounce portions)
Sausage, reduced-fat, hot/spicy
    Italian (separated into
    3-ounce portions)
Sausage, reduced-fat, mild
    Italian (separated into
    3-ounce portions)

Shrimp, shells on
Sole, fillet (frozen in 3-ounce
    portions)
Tilapia, fillet (frozen in 3-ounce
    portions)
Turkey, boneless breast or cutlet

Fats, Oils, Alcohol, and Sweets Group (use sparingly)

We prefer canola and olive oil because they have lower levels of saturated fat than other oils, such as sesame and corn oil. The alcohol we suggest stocking is intended for use in cooking and is used minimally to enhance the flavor of certain dishes, such as desserts and sauces. Alcohol should be used sparingly, and you should talk to your dietitian about how it might affect your meal plan.

Fats and Oils

Butter, unsalted
Coconut, unsweetened
    shredded
Cooking spray, canola oil based
Cooking spray, olive oil based

Margarine, liquid spray
Margarine, light solid
Oil, canola
Oil, olive
Oil, sesame

Sweets

Chocolate, semisweet baker's

Alcohol

Rum, dark
Rum, white
Tequila, light or dark
Wine, dry white, box or bottle
Wine, medium-dry red, box or bottle

Wine, Marsala
Sherry, cream
Sherry, dry
Vodka

Herbs, Spices, and Seasonings

Basil leaf, dried
Cayenne pepper, ground
Chili powder
Crushed red pepper flakes
Cumin, ground
Fennel seeds

Ground black pepper
Italian seasoning blend, no
    sodium
Marjoram, dried
Mustard, powdered
Oregano, dried

Paprika, ground
Parsley flakes, dried
Peppercorns, black and green
Rosemary, dried
Salt, iodized
Salt substitute
Sesame seeds
Thyme, dried
Sugar, confectioners'

Sugar, granulated (table sugar)
Sugar, granulated fructose (low-carbohydrate alternative)
Sweetener, Equal or NutraSweet
Sweetener, brown sugar alternative
Sweetener, Splenda Granular
Wasabi powder

Condiments

Chili paste
Dressings, low-fat or non-fat
Gravy Master
Hot sauce
Ketchup
Liquid Smoke

Mustard, Dijon
Mustard, spicy brown
Vinegar, balsamic
Vinegar, red wine
Vinegar, rice
Vinegar, white

Kitchen Equipment and Cooks' Tools

This section is broken down into general groups with brief comments about each particular item. You don't need to run out and buy everything on the list, and you don't need everything listed next to be able to prepare the recipes in this book. Having the items we mention, however, will make life in the kitchen easier and will expand your ability to prepare different things in different ways.

Hand Tools and Gadgets

Overall, look for durable, dishwasher-safe tools that you feel comfortable with. Cost does not necessarily equate with quality. You can find some very respectable kitchen tools at reasonable prices.

Meat mallet. Don't let the name fool you. In addition to pounding meat, meat mallets come in handy for crushing crackers, nuts, and more. Make sure you have one with a metal head, rather than wood, for easier, more effective cleaning.

Whisks. A fork comes through sometimes in a bind, but you have to have a few good whisks. Make sure you have a balloon whisk in addition to a rigid whisk.

Zester. One decent zester is all you'll ever need for getting perfect zest.

Vegetable peeler. Have at least two quality peelers on hand.

Kitchen shears. Another essential item that far too many people are without. Kitchen shears are used to cut through various food items, including meat. They should be sturdy, have stainless steel blades, and be dishwasher safe. A good set of kitchen shears is relatively inexpensive. They are also sometimes packaged with cutlery sets.

Spatulas. You should have at least three spatulas, preferably two flat plastic spatulas suitable for flipping or serving food from a pan, and one rubber spatula suitable for scraping food from bowls or pans. Heat-resistant rubber spatulas are worth the extra money. If you do any outdoor grilling, you may want to have a metal spatula as well.

Tongs. You should have at least three sets of metal tongs on hand for grilling, flipping, and picking up pieces of food. Have at least one long set of tongs for reaching into the oven or broiler with. Another reason to have more than one set is to avoid cross-contamination when cooking meat.

Cooking spoons. You should have several different types of long-handled spoons available to cook with, including slotted spoons. Wooden spoons are great because they don't scratch nonstick surfaces and they don't melt (but they can burn). Plastic spoons are also useful. Metal spoons are strong and durable.

Ladles. Have a few metal ladles, ranging in size from ½ ounce to 4 ounces. Ladles make measuring servings of sauces, soups, and other foods much easier.

Portion scoops. Similar to an ice cream scoop, these are great for portioning out muffin mix, rice, and other mixtures that require an exact size.

Measuring cups. Have two sets of dry measuring cups, preferably metal, and two liquid measuring cups, preferably in 1-cup and 4-cup sizes, with various measures marked off.

Measuring spoons. Have two or three sets of stainless steel, dishwasher-safe measuring spoons on hand. Don't ruin a recipe by "eyeballing" all your ingredients—nobody has an eye that good.

Cutting boards. Get yourself several dishwasher-safe, nonwood cutting boards. Wood cutting boards look nice, but they are more likely to harbor bacteria and can warp and crack over time. Choose only one or two large boards but make sure you have several smaller boards on hand. It is not uncommon to need two or three boards to prepare just one meal, especially if meat is involved.

Handheld graters. You should have at least one handheld grater, preferable with three sides of different grating sizes. Use it to quickly shred a carrot for a salad or to grate cheese. For big jobs, you should rely on a food processor.

Egg separator. As you will see, we are constantly calling for egg whites in our recipes. While you can shift an egg back and forth from half-shell to half-shell, having an egg separator sure makes life easier.

Thermometers. Cooking meats to the proper temperature is a very important aspect of food safety, reducing the risk of salmonella (poultry or meat), *E. coli* O157:H7 (raw or undercooked beef), and trichinosis (raw or undercooked pork and wild game). Spend about ten dollars on a decent meat thermometer and use it religiously. An oven thermometer is also worth having so you can check to make sure your oven is providing the right temperatures.

Kitchen scale. This should be an essential part of your kitchen, whether you have diabetes or not. You need to measure your portions for recipes as well as for adhering to serving sizes and your meal plan. There are plenty of dietary scales available that don't take up much counter space. Find one that has a detachable container on top or that has enough room for you to place a container on top with your food in it. Make sure you calibrate the scale to neutralize the weight of the container you use. By always using the same container for weighing your food, you won't have to keep changing the calibration (a small dish or custard cup usually works well). Be careful not to cross-contaminate your ingredients by weighing raw meat or eggs in the same container.

Salad spinner. You can use a strainer or colander to drain your lettuce after cleaning it, but what fun is that? Salad spinners quickly remove the water from greens, and you can get a decent one for very little money.

Cutlery

You can load your kitchen up with dozens of knives, but we think the following knives are essential and sufficient for most of your needs. Some of these knives are included in the standard knife block sets sold in department stores.

Chef's knife. Unless you plan on starring in a horror movie, keep the size of your chef's knife to between 8 and 10 inches.

Utility knife, 6- or 8-inch. An easy knife to handle, you'll use this all-purpose knife a lot for cutting vegetables and fruit.

Boning knife. The thin design of this knife makes it well suited for trimming fat and skin off poultry, which is highly suggested.

Paring knife. You should definitely have several paring knives on hand for all the little jobs that other knives are just too big for. Paring knives are usually between 2 and 4 inches long and have short handles.

Serrated bread knife. The only way to put an end to crushed bread is to use the right knife to slice it.

Pizza cutter. Besides being useful for slicing pizza, pizza cutters come in handy when working with dough. If you make our Baklava (page 193), then you'll see what we mean.

Minor Appliances

Food processor. A food processor on your counter will be used to perform a wide range of duties, including shredding, slicing, chopping, grinding, and puréeing. A good food processor should last a long time when properly cared for.

Electric stand mixer. This appliance takes care of things a food processor can't do. Electric mixers handle most baking tasks, from whipping eggs to mixing dough. The most popular models also offer attachments that expand the machine's functions, such as a pasta machine, a sausage maker, and a grater/shredder.

Electric blender. Blenders are well suited for liquids and are great for things like puréeing sauces, whipping dressings, and blending fruit smoothies. You can whip something up quickly and easily.

Microwave. In addition to reheating food and leftovers, microwaves are very useful for defrosting frozen food, such as meat, vegetables, broths, sauces, and fish. Microwaves are also great for cooking certain types of foods, including vegetables, rice, and some types of fish.

Toaster oven. Toaster ovens are great for baking, broiling, or toasting without having to heat a bigger oven. Not only do you save on energy use, but you also get the job done more quickly.

Electric hand mixer. Perfect for batters, cake mixes, and other baked goods, electric hand mixers are relatively inexpensive and should be a part of every kitchen.

Cookware

Nonstick skillets. Good sizes to have on hand range from 8 to 12 inches, with sloped and straight sides. Nonstick skillets reduce the need for fat in your stovetop cooking. Use them for everything from cooking eggs to sautéing onions. Choose skillets with riveted handles, if possible.

Stainless steel skillets. Choose skillets ranging from 6 to 12 inches. Make sure you get skillets that are oven-safe. Nonstick skillets are great, but stainless skillets are workhorses, perfect for everything from toasting seeds to simmering sauces. You can scrub them and use metal tools without worrying about the surface. Have both sloped-sided and straight-sided skillets. Choose skillets with riveted handles, if possible.

Pans. Pans have round sides and one long handle. Have a few different sizes available, preferably 1-quart, 2-quart, and 3-quart. In addition to making sauces, you'll use saucepans for steaming small portions of vegetables and for making smaller batches of soup. Choose pans with riveted handles, if possible.

Pots. Pots have straight sides and two handles, attached at opposite side of the rim. You should have a large stockpot and a smaller stockpot. Make sure one of them is big enough to cook pasta in. Choose pots with riveted handles, if possible.

Baking cookware. It is a good idea to have a few nonstick baking sheets, loaf pans, muffin pans, and baking pans in your cabinet. Nonstick cookware reduces or eliminates the need for adding fat when baking, and it also makes cleanup easier. Regular baking sheets are also good to have, especially for jobs that are best served by a more durable surface (like baking potatoes).

Steam baskets. Metal steam baskets sit inside a pot or saucepan, above boiling liquid, and hold the food you want to steam. Some people use bamboo baskets, especially for wok cooking, but we prefer the metal baskets. They are easier to clean and store and set right in the pot. We recommend that you have at least two metal steam baskets, a smaller one for vegetables and one large enough to fit a few portions of fish.

Colanders and strainers. You should have at least one steel colander with side handles and one plastic strainer with a straight handle. Steel colanders are great because they are strong and durable and well suited for heavy jobs, like straining chicken stock. A smaller, lighter plastic strainer is perfect for draining a few servings of pasta or rinsing fruits and vegetables. Also have on hand a small mesh strainer and a sieve. A China cap (a cone-shaped metal strainer) is great for straining stocks and can also be used to purée some foods.

Food mill. A food mill is used to purée and strain food at the same time. We use it when we prepare Nona's Italian Marinara Sauce (page 205).

Microwave rice steamer. An inexpensive rice steamer is one of the easiest ways to make perfectly steamed brown or white rice.

Miscellaneous

It may seem like we're stating the obvious here, but you might be surprised at how many people we find freezing foods in glass containers, using aluminum foil in the microwave or plastic wrap in the oven, or who still use a cereal bowl to combine recipe ingredients (what a mess).

Mixing bowls. You should have several mixing bowls of various sizes, ranging from small to large. Use for whisking, mixing, blending, tossing, and even serving. Use a big mixing bowl to soak lettuce to remove the dirt. Metal mixing bowls are a good choice because of their durability, but glass and ceramic bowls are generally microwave-safe and won't react with acidic foods such as tomatoes or marinades.

Storage containers. Select sturdy, dishwasher-safe containers that have tight-fitting lids. Have a few very small sizes, a few big sizes, and a whole bunch of sizes in the middle (1- to 4-cup containers are very practical). Try to use the same type so they can stack easily when being used or stored.

Resealable storage bags. Have at least two sizes, 1-quart and 1-gallon. Use the quart-size bags for leftovers, crushing walnuts or graham crackers, and marinating food. Use the bigger bags to store clean lettuce in so you can grab a handful for a salad. Freezer storage bags are good to have on hand because they reduce freezer burn.

Parchment paper. Parchment paper is an amazing product. Used to line a baking sheet or pan, it eliminates the need for greasing the pan. Whether you are baking cookies or latkes, the food just will not stick to it. Check the package for the exact temperature your parchment paper is safe for, but it is usually safe above 400 degrees F. You can find parchment paper in most supermarkets.

Aluminum foil. Essential for lining pans and cooking or wrapping food. It works very well in place of parchment paper when cooking *en papillote* because it can be easier to fold. Do not use aluminum foil, or any other metal, in the microwave.

Wax paper. Another essential found in most kitchens, although most people don't know what to use it for. We like it because it makes freezing meat and seafood easy. Use it to separate pieces of meat or fish before freezing and they will be easier to pull apart when you need just one piece. Wax paper is also great for handling or pressing sticky or crumbly food items, as we do when preparing our Key Lime Cheesecake Squares (page 191).

Plastic wrap. Just about everyone has this in their kitchen, and with good reason. Use it for wrapping food for storing and for defrosting food in the microwave.

Fire extinguisher. Even the most skilled cooks can have accidents in the kitchen. You should have a small fire extinguisher easily accessible to your kitchen. Better safe than sorry.

First aid kit. Make your own easy-access kit and keep it in your kitchen for emergencies. Include various size bandages, medical tape, gauze, and antiseptic. Also make sure you keep at least two pliable cold packs in your freezer.

3

Healthy Cooking Techniques

For a person living with diabetes, learning to use healthier cooking techniques is an important step in developing healthy eating habits. While making smart food choices is an essential element of meal planning and preparation, choosing smart cooking methods plays a huge role in defining what your finished product in the kitchen will be. Even the healthiest foods can be turned into a nutritional nightmare based solely on the way you cook them.

As you prepare recipes featured in *The Diabetic Gourmet Cookbook,* you will find that we use standard cooking methods as well as modified versions of standard methods in order to deliver dishes that are as healthy as they are delicious.

Some of our recipes are simply versions of traditional classics that have been cooked differently, such as our Grilled Chicken Parmesan over Penne (page 110). Traditionally, chicken parmesan is either fried in oil or sautéed in butter. We grill the chicken, which results in a much healthier dish that's actually easier to prepare.

We also use alternative techniques with the intention of simulating the results of less-healthy cooking methods. For example, in our recipe for Chicken Francese (page 107), the chicken is lightly breaded and baked, rather than being fried or sautéed in butter. Instead of using a butter-laden sauce, we use a broth-based sauce. The result is surprisingly similar to standard versions but is a much healthier dish.

The following methods are among the healthiest you can choose and are used throughout this cookbook. By familiarizing yourself with these cooking techniques and practicing them by preparing our recipes, you may be able to modify the preparation of other recipes to your nutritional benefit.

Steaming

One of the healthiest cooking techniques, steaming is cooking food over boiling water or other liquid. It requires no added oil or fat, it keeps food moist, and it retains most of the nutrients and flavor in the food.

Steaming food is easy. All you need to do is set the food in a metal steamer basket or rack in a pot over water (or some other liquid, like broth), bring the liquid to a boil, and cover the pot with a lid. The liquid level should reach just below the basket, so it doesn't actually touch the food. When steaming vegetables, steam until fork-tender. When steaming fish or meat, steam until cooked through.

Food can also be steamed quickly in the microwave using a similar method. Put a small amount of liquid into a microwave-safe bowl along with the food to be steamed, cover with a microwave-safe plate, and heat until the food is cooked to the degree you want. When using this method, the food cooks at the same time as the liquid boils, so you have to be careful not to overcook it. Try our Italian Summer Frittata (page 39) to see how we use the microwave to quickly steam fresh vegetables.

Grilling and Broiling

Grilling is cooking food directly over a heat source. Grilling is an especially good way to cook meat because it allows the fat to drip off. When using an outdoor grill, it is a good idea to wipe canola oil on the grill rack to help prevent food from sticking to it. Use a paper towel dipped in canola oil. Never spray a grill rack or open flame with nonstick cooking oil spray.

Broiling is similar to grilling, but the heat source is positioned above the food. Foods such as meat and poultry can be placed on a metal broiler pan that allows fat to drip away.

The degree of heat when grilling or broiling is generally determined by the distance between the food and the heat source, although the food is also cooked by the surrounding heat when broiling in an oven.

Grill pans have become increasingly popular over the past several years, and we call for their use frequently in this cookbook. A grill pan is a heavy pan with a rippled or ridged bottom. These ridges allow fat to run away from foods and also create sear marks on the food (like an outdoor grill). One of the best things about grill pans is that they are easy to use any time of the day and at any season of the year. Some of the recipes in this book that call for a grill pan include Grilled Chicken Parmesan over Penne (page 110), Tri-Colored Lemon Peppered Chicken (page 106), and Grilled Chicken Tostadas (page 108).

Pan-broiling involves cooking meat, poultry, or fish in a heavy skillet over medium-high to high heat without any added fat, oil, or other liquids. We use this technique for our Soho Sirloin Salad (page 85).

Baking and Roasting

When you bake or roast food, you surround the food with dry heat, which cooks it. Baking and roasting are basically the same technique, although the term "baking" is typically reserved for breads, starches, pastries, fruits, and fish, while "roasting" is used more often for meats.

We love to bake and roast, as you will see when you start preparing some of our recipes. One thing we especially enjoy doing is using the oven to "fry" food. By spraying a prepared food item, such as breaded chicken, with cooking spray, you can achieve the crisp texture of fried food without the added fat and calories.

Some recipes that require baking include Fiery Curry Tilapia (page 113), Sweet Potato Fries (page 167), Georgia Peach Pie (page 187), and Key Lime Cheesecake Squares (page 191). Recipes that require roasting include Classic Italian Meatballs in Pomodoro Sauce (page 132), Italian Roast Pork (page 137), and Roast Chicken with Black Raspberry Sauce (page 103).

Sautéing and Stir-Frying

Sautéing involves cooking food in a hot skillet with a small amount of fat, such as oil or butter. Stir-frying is basically the same thing, with a wok used instead of a skillet.

Our most frequently used method of sautéing, as you will see in many of our recipes, involves heating a nonstick skillet and then spraying it away from the heat source with nonstick canola spray. Using cooking spray helps reduce the overall fat content in many of our dishes without compromising the flavor and texture sautéing with added oil or fat provides. Sometimes a small amount of canola or olive oil is added to the skillet, but we do our best to use limited amounts. Some of the recipes requiring sautéing include Chicken Marsala (page 101) and Zucchini Sautéed with Garlic and Pepper (page 161). Recipes that are best prepared using a wok include Chicken and Cashew Stir-Fry (page 109) and Sesame Baby Bok Choy (page 153).

Poaching and Simmering

Cooking food in water or some other liquid, such as stock or wine, at a temperature below boiling (between 160 degrees F and 180 degrees F) is called poaching. Poaching requires no added fat, and it is a great choice for cooking certain foods, especially delicate foods. Foods suitable for poaching include poultry, fruit, fish, and eggs. A recipe that requires poaching in this book is Lemon-Poached Salmon (page 118).

Simmering is very similar to poaching, but the temperature of the liquid is higher (between 185 degrees F and 205 degrees F). Simmering is useful for tougher cuts of meat that require a long, moist cooking environment and for liquids that need to be reduced.

Foil Cooking or *En Papillote*

Foil cooking and cooking in paper *(en papillote)* require you to wrap food in aluminum foil or parchment paper so that it is sealed. The wrapped food is then heated in the oven, where it cooks in its own juices or a small amount of liquid that you may have added with the food. As the food cooks, the steam inside creates a moist environment that results in moist food. This method works very well for seafood, but can also be used for poultry. You have to be careful not to burn yourself with the steam when opening the wrapped food.

Braising and Stewing

Cooking food for a long period of time in an amount of liquid, covered, is known as braising or stewing. Braising usually involves a large piece of meat that is browned in some fat before being combined with liquid and cooked either on the stovetop or in the oven.

Stewing usually involves smaller pieces of food that are cooked or partially cooked before being combined with liquid and simmered. If a recipe asks you to brown meat in fat, we suggest coating your pot with nonstick cooking spray and just a small amount of canola oil.

A recipe that requires a slightly modified version of braising is Rustic Pot Roast with Vegetables (page 130), which uses cooking spray and a very small amount of fat to brown the meat. A recipe that mimics braising is Roast Cornish Game Hens in Sonoma Sauce (page 98), in which the hens are sprayed with cooking spray and roasted at high heat until browned on the outside.

4

Meal Planning

We mentioned earlier that the overall goal of diabetes treatment is to keep blood glucose levels as close to normal as possible. Meal planning is one of the most important tools for achieving this goal. The objective of meal planning is to keep your blood glucose levels as consistent as possible throughout the day through appropriate food choices and regularly scheduled meals.

A good meal plan should include a variety of different foods, including fruits, vegetables, grains, dairy, meat, and legumes, while taking individual nutritional requirements (and limitations) into consideration. Eating a variety of foods will not only make dining more interesting, but it also will help you get the nutrients your body needs for optimum health.

The major sources of energy from the foods you eat are fat, protein, and carbohydrate. Carbohydrate has the greatest effect on blood glucose levels, the amount depending on the type and quantity eaten, while fat and protein have a minimal effect. This is why diabetic meal planning focuses so heavily on carbohydrate intake. But while fat and protein don't have a great impact on glucose levels, their intake has to be closely regulated because of the negative effects they may have on your body (such as heart disease, high cholesterol, and kidney problems).

There are different approaches to meal planning, and it is important to choose the method that best suits your lifestyle and personal preferences. You should choose the method that is the easiest for you to understand and stick with. The more comfortable you are with the meal planning methods you choose, the more likely you are to be successful with your diet and diabetes management. Work closely with a dietitian or certified diabetes educator (CDE) until you have learned to follow a plan that works best for you. Revisit every several months to reevaluate your meal plan.

The two most popular methods for meal planning are known as Carbohydrate Counting and the Exchange Lists for Meal Planning. The recipes featured in this book and in *Diabetic Gourmet Magazine* provide the information needed to make appropriate food choices using either approach.

Just as the name implies, Carbohydrate Counting is based on counting the overall amount of carbohydrate you eat, whether they are starchy vegetables or cookies. Carbohydrate Counting is a popular meal planning choice because it offers a good level of flexibility when deciding what to eat. You can count carbohydrate based on the actual number of grams that are in the foods you eat.

Determining the amount of carbohydrate that a food contains can be difficult at times. Reading food labels, measuring ingredients when preparing your meals, and measuring the size of the servings you eat will help you control the amount of carbohydrate you are taking in. When preparing your own meals, you will need to read the food labels for the ingredients you are using. For food items without labels, such as meats, fruits, and vegetables, we suggest that you buy a book listing the nutritional information for a wide range of food items. Select a book that also includes the most commonly found dishes offered in restaurants so you can make smart choices when eating out. The United States Department of Agriculture Web site also offers a free, searchable food database that provides detailed nutritional information for thousands of food items. You can access the USDA Nutrient Database at http://www.nal.usda.gov/fnic/cgi-bin/nut_search.pl.

Most people use a core set of ingredients in their cooking and over time develop a good understanding of the foods they frequently use. One of the great things about a cookbook like this one is that the nutritional information and exchanges have already been calculated for you, making it easy to fit specific dishes into your meal plan. You simply choose a recipe based on your meal plan using the nutritional content or exchanges provided for the recipe, then follow the directions and adhere to the serving size. We provide a wide range of recipe types, including recipes that yield only one serving, and many of our recipes can be halved or doubled. This makes it easier to find a dish to prepare that fits your lifestyle and diet.

Exchange Lists for Meal Planning is a meal planning method developed by the American Dietetic Association and the American Diabetes

Association. It separates specific foods into categories to make it easier and faster to estimate the nutritional content of foods. Food items are given specific exchange values based on their nutritional content, mainly the amount of calories, fat, carbohydrate, and protein they contain, and are divided into lists of similar foods called exchange lists.

Exchange lists include starch/bread, meat, vegetable, fruit, milk/dairy, and fat. Food items in each exchange list are calculated so you can substitute one food item for another food item within the same list, provided you adhere to the serving sizes specified. For example, ½ cup cooked brown rice can be substituted for ½ cup cooked pasta. Food items in one list cannot be substituted for items that appear in a different list, regardless of the nutritional content. Your meal plan should contain foods from all the exchange lists each day to insure that you are eating a nutritionally balanced diet.

When using exchange lists for diabetic meal planning, you still have to measure ingredients and select foods that fit into your meal plan, but you won't have to spend as much time looking at carbohydrate and specific nutritional information when choosing foods. For more information about exchange lists, you can call the American Diabetes Association at 1-800-232-3472. You can find the most current exchange lists through your CDE or dietitan.

"Free foods" are foods and drinks that contain less than twenty calories. They usually do not need to be counted in meal planning when eaten in small amounts throughout the course of the day. Because many of these items are not completely free from calories and carbohydrate, they should be added to your meal plan calculations if an excessive amount has been eaten (or when free food amounts add up to a serving at one meal). Many vegetables, such as mushrooms, lettuce, spinach, cucumbers, and celery, are considered free foods, as are defatted broths, sugar-free sodas, and certain condiments such as mustard and vinegar.

Eating a variety of foods is an essential element of diabetes management and meal planning. The Diabetes Food Pyramid, as presented by the American Diabetes Association, is essentially an outline based on variety. It categorizes food items into several food groups along with the suggested number of daily servings that should be eaten from each group. It is very similar to the original Food Guide Pyramid designed by the United States Department of Agriculture, except for a few differences regarding some legumes and starchy vegetables.

Although you should still consult your dietitian for dietary recommendations suitable for you, the Food Guide Pyramid and the Diabetes

Food Pyramid are helpful tools in guiding your daily food choices. According to the Diabetes Food Pyramid, daily food intake should come from the following food groups.

Grains, Beans, and Starchy Vegetables (6 to 11 servings daily)

Select whole grain cereals, breads, and grains, such as brown rice, whole wheat bread, and oatmeal. Avoid foods high in fat or sugar, such as cakes and cookies. Foods in this group generally provide B vitamins, dietary fiber, iron, magnesium, and zinc. Studies show that a diet high in fiber may lower cholesterol levels, which could reduce the risk of heart disease. Legumes are a low-fat source of fiber that provides protein, folate, and other vitamins and minerals. If using canned legumes that contain sodium, rinse them under cool water.

Vegetable Group (3 to 5 servings daily)

You should eat a variety of vegetables each day, including dark green leafy vegetables and deep yellow vegetables. Steam, bake, roast, or grill vegetables for the best results. Vegetables can provide vitamin A, vitamin C, folate, magnesium, iron, and fiber.

Fruit Group (2 to 4 servings daily)

Select fresh fruit, frozen fruit with no added sugar, dried fruit, or canned fruit packed in water or natural juice instead of syrup. Fruits are a good source of vitamin A, vitamin C, potassium, and dietary fiber.

Milk Group (2 to 3 servings daily)

Choose low-fat and fat-free varieties of milk products and yogurt whenever possible. Milk is a good source of calcium, and fortified varieties offer vitamins A and D.

Meat and Other Group (2 to 3 servings daily)

Choose lean cuts of meat, skinless poultry, fish, tofu, and nuts. Trim fat from meat before cooking. Foods in this group are generally good sources of protein, niacin, iron, zinc, and vitamin B_{12}. Limit egg yolks because of cholesterol and fat, and limit nuts, which are also high in fat.

Fats, Oils, Alcohol, and Sweets Group (use sparingly)

Fats and oils should be used only in moderation, but they are essential elements in cooking and in our diets, and thus cannot be completely ignored. You should follow a diet low in saturated fat and cholesterol and moderate in total fat. Treats that are typically high in fat, sugar, calories, or cholesterol (such as candy, cookies, and regular soda) are considered sweets.

Meal planning requires you to become more involved with your eating than ever before. You're going to have to read food labels, measure ingredients when cooking, measure portions when serving, learn to say no, record how certain foods affect you, and eat at regularly scheduled times, and you must consult a professional (we can't stress this enough). It is also important to realize that your meal plan must be based on your individual needs, so what may be a good meal plan for someone else may not be good for you at all.

The American Diabetes Association recommends that people with diabetes contact a registered dietician to design a meal plan. To find a registered dietitian in your area who specializes in diabetes, call the American Dietetic Association at 1-800-366-1655, or visit http://www.eatright.com/find.html for a listing of dietitians based on your zip code. To find a diabetes educator in your area, call the American Association of Diabetes Educators at 1-800-TEAM-UP4. To find a diabetes education program in your area, call 1-800-DIABETES.

5

Breakfast and Brunch

It has often been said that breakfast is the most important meal of the day. This holds true for everyone, including people with diabetes. Some people are in such a hurry in the morning that they just ignore eating breakfast at home, opting instead to grab something on the road or to hold out until lunch. This is unfortunate because in a recent study, the American Heart Association reported that eating breakfast was associated with a 35 to 50 percent reduction in obesity and in insulin resistance, which can lead to heart disease and type 2 diabetes. Also, whole grain cereals have been found to reduce the risk for obesity and insulin resistance by as much as 15 percent.

If you have diabetes, then you probably already know how important it is to eat in the morning. It is also important that you make the right food choices. Many breakfast choices—such as muffins, doughnuts, and cakes—are high in calories, sugar, fat, cholesterol, and sodium and should be avoided. When it comes to fast food breakfast choices, the best choice is to just keep driving.

Try to select whole grain cereals, breads, and grains, such as whole wheat bread and oatmeal. Our French Toast for Two, prepared using whole wheat bread and egg whites, is low in cholesterol, fat, and sugar and high in fiber. Whole grain cereals, breads, and grains provide B vitamins, iron, complex carbohydrate, and dietary fiber. Studies show that a diet high in fiber may lower cholesterol levels, which could reduce the risk of heart disease. For your breakfast cereals, choose low-fat and fat-free milk products, like skim milk and low-fat yogurt. If you want more of a sweet treat for breakfast, then try our Cranberry Scones, Blueberry Buttermilk Pancakes, or Chocolate Chip Pancakes.

Everybody seems busy these days. That's why we've included several breakfast recipes that are quick and easy to prepare, such as Soy Yogurt Smoothie, Breakfast Berry Parfait, Warm Scottish Oatmeal with Cranberries, and Hawaiian Sunrise. When selecting fruit, choose fresh fruit, frozen fruit with no added sugar, dried fruit, or canned fruit packed in water or natural juice instead of syrup. Fruit is a good source of vitamin A, vitamin C, potassium, and dietary fiber and is good to include at breakfast.

If you find that you have a few extra minutes in the morning, then cook up an Italian Summer Frittata or Open-Faced Omelet Florentine using one of our egg mixes. Saturdays and Sundays are especially good for our eye-opening Huevos Rancheros or freshly baked Cinnamon Buns because they take a little extra time to prepare.

Brunch—that delightful cross between breakfast and lunch—is most often enjoyed on the weekends. While many people believe brunch is an American creation, it actually sprang up in England in the early 1900s. When we think of brunch, we think of a prolonged, more social meal that can include dishes people don't usually get a chance to eat on the busy weekdays. Some good brunch dishes include Spinach and Feta Quiche, Pecan Winter Waffles, Smoked Salmon Bagel with Dill-Chive Spread, Latkes with Smoked Salmon, and Blueberry Blintzes Topped with Lime Crema. These recipes are especially well suited for brunch because of their expandability and appealing presentation.

Latkes with Smoked Salmon

Latkes, or potato pancakes, are a traditional Jewish dish often served at holidays. This version adds smoked salmon and a light chive topping. It makes for a stimulating breakfast or brunch dish that is low in fat and cholesterol.

1½ pounds potatoes, peeled
½ cup finely chopped yellow onion
1 tablespoon all-purpose flour
3 egg whites
4 teaspoons chopped chives, divided
½ teaspoon salt substitute
⅛ teaspoon freshly ground black pepper
Canola cooking spray
½ cup fat-free sour cream
6 ounces thinly sliced smoked salmon

Preheat oven to 400 degrees F.

Grate the potatoes using a food processor. Soak in cold water for 10 minutes, then remove to a colander and drain well. Using a towel, squeeze as much of the water out of the potatoes as possible.

Place the potatoes in a large mixing bowl and add the onion, flour, egg whites, 2 teaspoons chives, salt substitute, and black pepper. Stir until well combined.

Line a baking sheet with parchment paper, or spray heavily with cooking spray. Shape the potato mixture into 3-inch round cakes and arrange on the baking sheet so they are not touching.

Spray the latkes lightly with cooking spray and bake for 10 minutes, or until the tops of the latkes become golden. Flip each latke over and spray lightly with cooking spray. Bake for another 15 to 20 minutes, or until golden brown.

Meanwhile, combine the sour cream and remaining 2 teaspoons chives in a small bowl. Refrigerate until ready to use.

Divide the baked latkes among 6 plates. Top each with 1 ounce smoked salmon and about 1 tablespoon sour cream topping.

YIELD: 6 servings, 3 3-inch latkes per serving

Nutritional Information Per Serving (3 latkes plus 1 ounce of salmon):

Calories: 144
Fat: 1.3 g
  Saturated Fat: 0.3 g
  Monounsaturated Fat: 0.6 g
  Polyunsaturated Fat: 0.4 g
Cholesterol: 8 mg
Sodium: 280 mg
Carbohydrate: 22.9 g
Dietary Fiber: 1.9 g
Sugars: 3.1 g
Starches: 14.3 g
Protein: 9.9 g
Diabetic Exchanges:
  1½ Bread/Starch, ½ Fat

Home Fries

We suggest that you cook the potatoes the night before and cut them in the morning once they are fully cooled. Some people like fresh minced garlic added to their home fries. If you want to include garlic, add it to the skillet when you add the cut potatoes to the onion.

YIELD: 4 servings

**Nutritional Information
Per Serving (½ cup):**
Calories: 179
Fat: 1.9 g
  Saturated Fat: 0.2 g
  Monounsaturated Fat: 0.7 g
  Polyunsaturated Fat: 0.8 g
Cholesterol: 0 mg
Sodium: 15 mg
Carbohydrate: 38.1 g
Dietary Fiber: 3.9 g
Sugars: 2.5 g
Starches: 0.3 g
Protein: 3.8 g
Diabetic Exchanges:
  2½ Starch/Bread

10 small new potatoes, scrubbed, skins left on
  (about 1 pound)
1 teaspoon canola oil
1 medium sweet onion, diced
1 teaspoon light margarine
1 teaspoon paprika, or more to taste
¼ teaspoon freshly ground black pepper, or to taste
⅛ teaspoon salt, optional

Bring a large pot of water to a boil. Add the potatoes and cook for 9 to 12 minutes, or until fork tender. Drain and rinse under cold water. Once the potatoes have cooled off, cut each one in half. Measure out 2 cups of potatoes.

Meanwhile, heat the canola oil in a large non-stick skillet over medium-low heat. Add the diced onion and sauté until softened and golden brown, about 7 minutes.

Add the cut potatoes and margarine to the sautéed onion; turn the heat up to medium. Sprinkle with the paprika, black pepper, and salt. Cook, stirring frequently, until the potatoes are well heated, about 5 minutes.

Buttermilk Waffles

This recipe requires a waffle iron. Decent electric waffle irons are readily available in most department stores for as little as ten dollars and are easy to use. This waffle batter will keep for up to three days, covered and refrigerated. Just whisk it briefly before using. Instead of syrup, try one of these optional toppings per serving: fresh berries or fruit, fat-free nondairy whipped topping, sugar-free chocolate syrup.

YIELD: 6 servings, 1 waffle per serving

Nutritional Information Per Serving (1 waffle):
Calories: 241
Fat: 6.2 g
  Saturated Fat: 0.8 g
  Monounsaturated Fat: 2.4 g
  Polyunsaturated Fat: 2.4 g
Cholesterol: 37 mg
Sodium: 416 mg
Carbohydrate: 36.7 g
Dietary Fiber: 2.1 g
Sugars: 4.5 g
Starches: 1.1 g
Protein: 9.6 g
Diabetic Exchanges:
  2½ Starch/Bread, 1 Fat

1 egg
2 egg whites
1½ cups all-purpose flour
½ cup whole wheat flour
1 teaspoon granulated sugar
4 teaspoons baking powder
¼ teaspoon salt
2 tablespoons canola oil
1¾ cups nonfat skim milk
¼ cup low-fat buttermilk
½ teaspoon pure vanilla extract
Canola cooking spray
Sugar-free pancake syrup

Preheat waffle iron.

In a small bowl, whisk the egg and egg whites until fluffy.

In a large bowl, whisk together the flours, sugar, baking powder, and salt. Beat in the eggs, canola oil, skim milk, buttermilk, and vanilla until smooth.

Lightly spray heated waffle iron with cooking spray. Pour ⅔ cup batter into the waffle iron; close the iron and cook until waffle is golden brown.

Serve hot with sugar-free pancake syrup.

Pecan Winter Waffles

This recipe requires a waffle iron. Decent electric waffle irons are readily available in most department stores for as little as ten dollars and are easy to use. These flavorful waffles can be a real hit on a cold winter day, and they are easy to make. The batter will keep overnight, covered and refrigerated. Just whisk it briefly before using.

YIELD: 8 servings, 1 waffle per serving

Nutritional Information Per Serving (1 waffle):
Calories: 214
Fat: 7.5 g
  Saturated Fat: 1.2 g
  Monounsaturated Fat: 3.2 g
  Polyunsaturated Fat: 2.5 g
Cholesterol: 55 mg
Sodium: 443 mg
Carbohydrate: 28.4 g
Dietary Fiber: 2.0 g
Sugars: 4.1 g
Starches: 0.1 g
Protein: 8.4 g
Diabetic Exchanges:
  2 Starch/Bread, 1½ Fat

1½ teaspoons active dry yeast
2 tablespoons warm water
1½ cups all-purpose flour
½ cup whole wheat flour
2 teaspoons granulated sugar
½ teaspoon salt
1 teaspoon baking soda
1 teaspoon baking powder
½ teaspoon ground cinnamon
Pinch ground nutmeg
2 eggs
2 egg whites
2 cups low-fat buttermilk
2 tablespoons canola oil
½ teaspoon pure vanilla extract
Canola cooking spray
8 teaspoons chopped pecans
Sugar-free pancake syrup, optional

Preheat waffle iron.

In a small bowl, stir yeast into the water and set aside for 10 minutes.

In a large bowl, combine the flours, sugar, salt, baking soda, baking powder, cinnamon, and nutmeg.

Add the eggs, egg whites, buttermilk, oil, vanilla, and yeast mixture; whisk until smooth.

Lightly spray the heated waffle iron with cooking spray. Pour ⅔ cup batter into the waffle iron. Once the batter is in the iron, sprinkle with 1 teaspoon chopped pecans. Close the waffle iron and cook until waffle is golden brown.

Serve hot with sugar-free pancake syrup, if desired.

Blueberry Buttermilk Pancakes

One of the best tips we can give you about making pancakes is that you should flip a pancake only once. Patience is essential, so make sure you wait until bubbles form on the top of the pancake, or the bottom becomes golden, before you flip. Once you flip the pancake, allow it to cook through and then take it off the heat. If you keep flipping a pancake over and over, it will become dense.

1¼ cups all-purpose flour
½ teaspoon granulated sugar
¼ teaspoon salt
1¼ teaspoons baking powder
1¼ cups low-fat buttermilk
2 tablespoons water
1 egg
1 egg white
Canola cooking spray
¾ cup fresh or frozen blueberries, thawed if frozen
Sugar-free pancake syrup, optional

In a large bowl, combine the flour, sugar, salt, and baking powder.

In another large bowl, whisk the buttermilk, water, egg, and egg white.

Gradually add the flour mixture to the buttermilk mixture, whisking until well combined. Let stand for 5 minutes.

Heat a large nonstick griddle or skillet over medium-high heat until hot. Move the griddle or skillet away from the heat source, lightly spray with cooking spray, and return to the heat.

For each pancake, pour ⅓ cup batter on the griddle and immediately sprinkle 5 or 6 blueberries into the pancake. Cook until bubbles form on the top of the pancake, or until the bottom of the pancake turns golden, about 40 seconds. Flip the pancake over and cook for another 25 to 30 seconds, or until cooked through.

Serve the pancakes while they are still hot. You can top them with some sugar-free pancake syrup if you wish, but they are plenty sweet and tasty all by themselves.

YIELD: 4 servings, 2 6-inch pancakes per serving

Nutritional Information Per Serving (2 pancakes):

Calories: 214
Fat: 2.4 g
  Saturated Fat: 0.8 g
  Monounsaturated Fat: 0.7 g
  Polyunsaturated Fat: 0.4 g
Cholesterol: 56 mg
Sodium: 371 mg
Carbohydrate: 38.4 g
Dietary Fiber: 1.8 g
Sugars: 6.2 g
Starches: 1.5 g
Protein: 9.2 g
Diabetic Exchanges:
  2½ Starch/Bread, ½ Fat

Fruit Pancake Variations

Substitute chunks or slices of fruit about the size of a small blueberry for the blueberries used in each pancake. If you add pieces that are bigger than a blueberry, you might run into problems getting the pancake to cook properly. Good fruit choices include bananas and strawberries.

Chocolate Chip Pancakes

For a real chocolate fest, add two teaspoons of sugar-free chocolate syrup (or more to taste) when you whisk in the milk or just drizzle some over the pancakes when they are ready to serve.

1½ cups all-purpose flour
½ teaspoon granulated sugar
1½ teaspoons baking powder
¼ teaspoon salt
1¼ cups skim milk
¼ cup evaporated skim milk
3 tablespoons water
1 large egg
2 egg whites
½ teaspoon pure vanilla extract
Canola cooking spray
2 tablespoons semisweet chocolate chips
Sugar-free pancake syrup, optional
Light nondairy whipped topping, optional

YIELD: 4 servings, 2 6-inch pancakes per serving

Nutritional Information Per Serving (2 pancakes):

Calories: 247
Fat: 2.9 g
 Saturated Fat: 1.1 g
 Monounsaturated Fat: 0.9 g
 Polyunsaturated Fat: 0.4 g
Cholesterol: 55 mg
Sodium: 367 mg
Carbohydrate: 43.1 g
Dietary Fiber: 1.5 g
Sugars: 6.1 g
Starches: 0.8 g
Protein: 11 g
Diabetic Exchanges:
 3 Starch/Bread, ½ Fat

In a large mixing bowl, whisk together the flour, sugar, baking powder, and salt.

In a medium bowl, whisk together the skim milk, evaporated skim milk, water, egg, egg whites, and vanilla.

Gradually add the wet ingredients to the dry ingredients, whisking until well combined and smooth. Let stand for 5 minutes.

Heat a large nonstick griddle or skillet over medium-high heat until hot. Move the griddle or skillet away from the heat source, lightly spray with cooking spray, and return to the heat.

For each pancake, pour ⅓ cup batter on the griddle and immediately push 5 or 6 chocolate chips into the pancake. Cook until bubbles form on the top of the pancake, or until the bottom of the pancake turns golden, about 40 seconds. Flip the pancake over and cook for another 25 to 30 seconds, or until cooked through.

Serve the pancakes while they are still hot. You can top them with some sugar-free pancake syrup or a dollop of light nondairy whipped topping if you wish (not included in nutritional information).

Fruit Pancake Variations

Substitute small pieces of fruit for the chocolate chips. Good fruit choices include blueberries, bananas, and strawberries.

French Toast for Two

How is it that something so tasty and simple to make is so often forgotten? You can get a hot, delicious serving of French toast on the table in just about 10 minutes, and it's something the whole family can enjoy. This recipe can be doubled easily.

4 egg whites
¼ cup evaporated skim milk
⅛ cup skim milk
¼ teaspoon ground cinnamon
⅛ teaspoon ground nutmeg
¼ teaspoon vanilla extract
Canola cooking spray
6 slices reduced-calorie whole wheat bread
Sugar-free pancake syrup, optional
Fresh berries, optional

In a medium bowl, whisk together the egg whites, evaporated skim milk, skim milk, cinnamon, nutmeg, and vanilla until well blended.

Heat a large nonstick griddle or skillet over medium heat until hot. Away from the heat source, spray lightly with cooking spray, and return to the heat.

Dip each slice of bread into the egg mixture so that both sides are evenly coated. Place on the

YIELD: 2 servings, 3 pieces per serving

Nutritional Information Per Serving (3 pieces):

Calories: 204
Fat: 1.7 g
  Saturated Fat: 0.3 g
  Monounsaturated Fat: 0.2 g
  Polyunsaturated Fat: 0.7 g
Cholesterol: 2 mg
Sodium: 508 mg
Carbohydrate: 35.6 g
Dietary Fiber: 8.5 g
Sugars: 1.5 g
Starches: 0.1 g
Protein: 16.3 g
Diabetic Exchanges: 2 Starch/Bread, ½ Fat-Free Milk

griddle and cook for 60 to 90 seconds on each side, or until both sides become golden.

Serve hot with sugar-free pancake syrup or fresh fruit (not included in nutritional analysis).

Cholesterol-Free Egg Mix

Here is a great way to enjoy cholesterol-free, fat-free eggs without having to resort to store-bought mixtures that can contain things you've never heard of and cost a fortune over time. If you are on a cholesterol-restricted diet, then this is the egg mix for you. If you are not necessarily on a cholesterol-restricted diet, then you may prefer Our Basic Egg Mix (recipe follows), which holds up better during cooking.

9 egg whites
2 tablespoons water
5 drops yellow food coloring, optional

Combine all the ingredients in a large bowl and whisk until frothy and well blended.

Refrigerate in a container, covered, for up to 1 week.

YIELD: 1 cup, 3 (⅓ cup) servings

Nutritional Information Per Serving (⅓ cup):
Calories: 51
Fat: 0 g
  Saturated Fat: 0 g
  Monounsaturated Fat: 0 g
  Polyunsaturated Fat: 0 g
Cholesterol: 0 mg
Sodium: 165 mg
Carbohydrate: 1 g
Dietary Fiber: 0 g
Sugars: 1 g
Starches: 0 g
Protein: 10.5 g
Diabetic Exchanges: 1½ Very
  Lean Meat

Our Basic Egg Mix

This is our low-cholesterol, low-fat egg mix. It is versatile enough to be used for almost every recipe that calls for regular eggs, including omelets. Unlike our cholesterol-free version, this mix maintains the texture and stability of whole eggs much better.

9 egg whites
1 egg
2 tablespoons water
1 or 2 drops yellow food coloring, optional

Combine all the ingredients in a large bowl and whisk until well blended.

Refrigerate in a container, covered, for up to 1 week.

YIELD: 1 cup, 3 (⅓ cup) servings

Nutritional Information Per Serving (⅓ cup):
Calories: 76
Fat: 1.7 g
  Saturated Fat: 0.5 g
  Monounsaturated Fat: 0.6 g
  Polyunsaturated Fat: 0.2 g
Cholesterol: 71 mg
Sodium: 186 mg
Carbohydrate: 1.3 g
Dietary Fiber: 0 g
Sugars: 1.0 g
Starches: 0 g
Protein: 12.6 g
Diabetic Exchanges: 1½ Very
  Lean Meat

Western Omelet with Cheese

A perennial diner favorite across the United States, the Western omelet can be found in a number of different variations. Our version is simple to prepare and lower in fat, calories, and cholesterol.

1 teaspoon canola oil
¼ cup chopped yellow onion
¼ cup chopped green bell pepper
1 slice 97% fat-free, low-sodium ham, about 1 ounce, chopped
Pinch ground black pepper
Canola cooking spray
⅓ cup Our Basic Egg Mix (page 37) or Cholesterol-Free Egg Mix (page 37) or egg substitute
1 ounce shredded low-sodium, reduced-fat Cheddar cheese

YIELD: 1 serving

Nutritional Information Per Serving:

Calories: 173
Fat: 4.9 g
  Saturated Fat: 2.2 g
  Monounsaturated Fat: 1.7 g
  Polyunsaturated Fat: 0.5 g
Cholesterol: 85 mg
Sodium: 330 mg
Carbohydrate: 7.7 g
Dietary Fiber: 1.4 g
Sugars: 1.0 g
Starches: 0 g
Protein: 23.4 g
Diabetic Exchanges:
  1 Medium-Fat Meat, 3 Vegetable

Heat an 8-inch nonstick skillet over medium heat. Away from the heat source, coat the pan with cooking spray. Return to the heat, add the onion and pepper, and sauté until onion softens, about 5 minutes. Stir in the chopped ham and black pepper and heat for 1 minute. Remove mixture to a small bowl.

Away from the heat source, lightly spray the skillet with cooking spray again and return to the heat. Pour the egg mix into the skillet and swirl the skillet around until the mixture covers the entire pan. Allow to cook for 30 seconds, or until the eggs have become firm and cooked around the edges.

Using a spatula, loosen the eggs from the sides of the skillet and carefully flip it over. Sprinkle with the shredded cheese. Spoon the ham and vegetable mixture into the center of the egg mixture and spread it out across the width of the omelet. Use the spatula to fold the omelet over until the edges meet, forming a semicircle. Reduce the heat to low and cook for another 30 seconds, or until the cheese is melted. Slide the omelet onto a plate and serve hot.

Italian Summer Frittata

A frittata is an open-faced omelet that is often finished in the oven, which lends it a fluffier consistency. This very colorful frittata provides a wonderful range of flavors and textures, and it makes a great dish for breakfast or brunch.

1 small green zucchini, sliced into ⅛-inch slices (about 1 cup)
½ cup chopped sweet yellow onion, such as Vidalia
2 tablespoons water
1½ cups Our Basic Egg Mix (page 37) or egg substitute
2 tablespoons sliced scallion, green part only
¼ teaspoon salt-free Italian seasoning
Canola cooking spray
8 grape tomatoes, or 4 cherry tomatoes cut in half
Dash black pepper
½ cup chopped roasted red pepper
2 tablespoons grated Parmesan cheese
1 teaspoon fresh chopped parsley, optional garnish

YIELD: 4 servings

Nutritional Information Per Serving (¼ of recipe):
Calories: 114
Fat: 2.9 g
 Saturated Fat: 1.2 g
 Monounsaturated Fat: 0.9 g
 Polyunsaturated Fat: 0.3 g
Cholesterol: 73 mg
Sodium: 335 mg
Carbohydrate: 6.4 g
Dietary Fiber: 1.4 g
Sugars: 2.3 g
Starches: 0 g
Protein: 15.1 g
Diabetic Exchanges: 2 Very Lean Meat, 2 Vegetable

Preheat broiler.

Place the zucchini, onion, and water in a microwave-safe dish. Cover with a microwave-safe plate and heat for 3 minutes, or until the zucchini is fork tender.

Whisk together the egg, scallion, and Italian seasoning.

Heat a 10-inch oven-safe nonstick skillet over medium heat. Away from the heat source, spray with cooking spray. Return to the heat, add the egg mixture, and cook until almost set.

Scatter the cooked vegetables, tomatoes, and roasted red pepper over the egg. Season lightly with black pepper and sprinkle with grated cheese. Set the entire skillet under the hot broiler until the egg is cooked and cheese has melted. Place on a large plate and cut into 4 wedges (like a pizza). Garnish with fresh parsley, if desired, and serve.

Open-Faced Omelet Florentine

Many of us eat breakfast solo, which can make recipes for two or more people a problem. This is the perfect one-person breakfast dish. It's simple to make and you should be able to get it on the table in less than 10 minutes. You can use ⅓ cup of our Cholesterol-Free Egg Mix (page 37) or Our Basic Egg Mix (page 37) instead of the eggs and water called for in this recipe.

1 egg
3 egg whites
1 teaspoon water
1 tablespoon thinly sliced scallions, green part only
1 cup packed fresh spinach leaves
¾ ounce shredded reduced-fat mild Cheddar cheese
1 tablespoon sliced basil leaves
Canola cooking spray
4 ¼-inch thick tomato slices

YIELD: 1 serving

Nutritional Information Per Serving:

Calories: 189
Fat: 6.9 g
  Saturated Fat: 2.3 g
  Monounsaturated Fat: 2.4 g
  Polyunsaturated Fat: 0.9 g
Cholesterol: 217 mg
Sodium: 391 mg
Carbohydrate: 7.3 g
Dietary Fiber: 1.9 g
Sugars: 1.5 g
Starches: 0.1 g
Protein: 23.7 g
Diabetic Exchanges: 3 Very
  Lean Meat, 2 Vegetable,
  1 Fat

Whisk together the eggs, egg whites, water, and scallions in a mixing bowl.

Place the spinach leaves in a microwave-safe bowl and cover with a microwave-safe dish. Heat for 30 to 45 seconds, or until the spinach is hot and somewhat wilted.

In a small bowl, toss the shredded cheese with the sliced basil until well combined.

Heat an 8-inch nonstick skillet over medium heat until hot. Away from the heat source, spray with cooking spray and add the egg mixture. Return to the heat and cook the egg mixture until almost set, pulling in the edges with a spatula as it cooks to allow uncooked egg to reach the skillet.

Flip the entire egg over carefully to keep it in one piece. Spread the tomato slices on top of the egg and scatter the spinach leaves over it. Sprinkle with the shredded cheese mixture, cover, and turn off the heat. Allow to sit for 1 minute, covered, or until the cheese softens and melts a little bit before serving.

Huevos Rancheros

Talk about starting off the day with a bang! This dish is basically poached eggs in a loose tomato salsa. But when all is said and done, this presents well, tastes great, and adds some excitement to the day. This recipe can be doubled, but you must divide the ingredients and prepare each serving in its own skillet. If you need to reduce the amount of cholesterol, replace the whole egg with 1 egg white for an equally satisfying dish.

YIELD: 1 serving

Nutritional Information Per Serving:

Calories: 317
Fat: 8.2 g
  Saturated Fat: 3.3 g
  Monounsaturated Fat: 2.7 g
  Polyunsaturated Fat: 1.3 g
Cholesterol: 220 mg
Sodium: 268 mg
Carbohydrate: 37 g
Dietary Fiber: 5.9 g
Sugars: 5.0 g
Starches: 10.6 g
Protein: 26 g
Diabetic Exchanges:
  1 Starch/Bread, 2 Very Lean Meat, 4 Vegetable, 1 Fat

Canola cooking spray
1 6-inch corn tortilla
Salt substitute
½ cup chopped yellow onion
1 tablespoon minced garlic
1 cup canned low-sodium diced tomatoes, including juice
½ cup water
Dash chili powder
Dash hot pepper sauce
4 slices pickled jalapeño pepper rings, or more to taste
Pinch dried oregano
Pinch ground black pepper
1 egg
2 egg whites
¼ cup shredded reduced-fat, low-sodium Cheddar cheese
¼ cup shredded iceberg lettuce
2 teaspoons fat-free sour cream
1 tablespoon sliced scallions, green part only

Preheat oven to 425 degrees F.

Line a baking sheet with aluminum foil and spray lightly with cooking spray. Lightly spray the tortilla with cooking spray. Place on the baking sheet and bake for 5 to 7 minutes, flipping once, or until crisp. Remove to a paper towel, sprinkle with salt substitute, and set aside.

Meanwhile, heat an 8-inch or 10-inch nonstick skillet over medium heat. Away from the heat source, heavily coat with cooking spray and return to the heat. Sauté the onion until softened, about

5 minutes. Add the garlic and sauté for 1 minute. Add the tomatoes, water, chili powder, hot sauce, jalapeño pepper rings, oregano, and black pepper; cover and simmer for 5 minutes, stirring occasionally.

Place the egg and the egg whites in a small bowl, being careful not to break the yolk. Slowly pour the eggs, all at once, into the center of the simmering tomato mixture. Cover and simmer for 5 minutes, or until the egg is just about set. Sprinkle the entire mixture with shredded cheese and cover. Simmer until the cheese is completely melted.

Carefully slide the contents of the skillet onto a large dinner plate. Place the crisp tortilla to the side, tucked slightly under the edge of the huevos rancheros. Pile the shredded lettuce beside the tortilla and top with sour cream. Sprinkle the entire dish with scallions and serve at once.

Spinach and Feta Quiche

Quiche is another dish that people seem to forget about, which is a shame considering how easy it can be to make. This version pairs the classic combination of spinach and feta cheese and gets a nice addition of color from the red pepper. Leftovers reheat well in the microwave, but be careful not to overheat them.

1 9-inch frozen reduced-fat pie shell
Canola cooking spray
¾ cup chopped yellow onion
1 clove garlic, minced
1 10-ounce package frozen chopped spinach, thawed, drained, excess liquid squeezed out
2 tablespoons chopped roasted red pepper
½ cup crumbled feta cheese
1 egg
3 egg whites
⅓ cup fat-free milk
½ cup evaporated skim milk
¼ teaspoon ground dried oregano
Pinch ground black pepper

YIELD: 8 servings, 1 slice per serving

Nutritional Information Per Serving (1 slice):
Calories: 192
Fat: 9.8 g
 Saturated Fat: 3.2 g
 Monounsaturated Fat: 3.7 g
 Polyunsaturated Fat: 0.2 g
Cholesterol: 35 mg
Sodium: 321 mg
Carbohydrate: 19.9 g
Dietary Fiber: 1.4 g
Sugars: 5.3 g
Starches: 0.5 g
Protein: 8.3 g
Diabetic Exchanges:
 ½ Starch/Bread, 1 Vegetable,
 ½ Reduced-Fat Milk, 1½ Fat

Sugar Free, Assorted

NUTRITION FACTS

Serving Size: 3 Pieces (40g)

Amount Per Serving

Calories 170   Calories from Fat 80

	% Daily Value*
Total Fat 10g	15%
Saturated Fat 6g	30%
Cholesterol < 5mg	1%
Sodium 10mg	0%
Total Carbohydrates 14g	5%
Dietary Fiber < 1g	2%
Sugars 0g	0%
Sugar Alcohols 11g	
Protein 1g	

Vitamin A 0%	Vitamin C 0%
Calcium 0%	Iron 0%

*Percent Daily Values are based on a 2,000 calorie diet. Your daily value may be higher or lower depending on your caloric needs.

SUGAR FREE

- Our Sugar Free containers now contain MALTITOL, derived from corn, non-cariogenic (does not promote tooth decay).

- Excess consumption may have a laxative effect, therefore we recommend that daily consumption for adults be limited to approximately 50 grams (about 1 ¾ oz.) or about 4 pieces.

- This candy contains the same number of calories as sugar based candy and is not dietetic. It may be useful in the diet of a diabetic person on the advice of a physician.

- Not a reduced calorie product.
- No salt added.

Chocolate Sparrow
5 Old Colony Way
Orleans, MA 02653
1-800-922-6399
508-240-6970

Preheat oven to 375 degrees F.

Bake the pie shell for 15 minutes, or until it just begins to turn golden. Remove from oven and set aside.

Meanwhile, heat a large nonstick skillet over medium heat. Away from the heat source, spray with cooking spray and return to the heat. Sauté the onion until softened, about 5 minutes. Add the garlic and sauté for 1 minute. Add the spinach and roasted pepper and heat for 1 minute, stirring until heated and excess water from the spinach is cooked off. Remove from the heat and stir in the feta cheese until well combined; set aside.

In a large bowl, whisk the egg, egg whites, milk, evaporated milk, oregano, and black pepper.

Spoon the spinach mixture into the pie shell and spread out into an even layer.

Ladle the egg mixture into the pie shell, pouring it directly over the spinach, until it fills the shell, just reaching the lower lip of the pie shell's inner rim. Depending on the pie shell you have, you may have leftover egg mixture, which you can discard (don't use it to overfill your quiche).

Place on a baking sheet and bake on the middle oven rack for 35 to 40 minutes, or until the quiche is just set. Remove from the oven and allow to cool for about 10 minutes. Cut into 8 slices, like a pie, and serve while warm.

Leftover quiche can keep for 2 to 3 days, refrigerated and covered, and should last a few weeks if frozen. Reheat individual slices in the microwave until hot, or reheat in the oven at 350 degrees F until hot in the center.

Smoked Salmon Bagel with Dill-Chive Spread

Resembling scallions, chives have a mild onion flavor that complements many dishes, including dressings, sauces, and spreads. The smoked salmon adds quite a bit of sodium to this dish, so make sure it fits in with your meal plan. This recipe easily doubles and is great for breakfast or brunch.

2 teaspoons fat-free sour cream
1 teaspoon light or fat-free cream cheese
½ teaspoon chopped fresh dill, or ¼ teaspoon dried dill
1 teaspoon chopped chives plus extra for garnish
½ sesame seed bagel (pumpernickel, jalapeño, plain, or whole wheat bagels also work well)
1 leaf green leaf lettuce
2 thin slices tomato
6 thin strips (about 2½ ounces) smoked salmon

In a small bowl, mix the sour cream, cream cheese, dill, and chives until well blended. Spread the mixture on the bagel half. Top with lettuce leaf, tomato slices, and salmon and serve sprinkled with the extra chives, if desired.

YIELD: 1 serving

Nutritional Information Per Serving:
Calories: 180
Fat: 3.6 g
 Saturated Fat: 0.7 g
 Monounsaturated Fat: 1.5 g
 Polyunsaturated Fat: 0.9 g
Cholesterol: 18 mg
Sodium: 743 mg
Carbohydrate: 19.1 g
Dietary Fiber: 2.7 g
Sugars: 0.8 g
Starches: 0.5 g
Protein: 17.9 g
Diabetic Exchanges:
 1 Starch/Bread, 1 Medium-Fat Meat

Breakfast Berry Parfait

You can use blackberries, blueberries, or raspberries instead of strawberries, or a mix of all three. This parfait will keep overnight, refrigerated, so you can make it ahead of time for breakfast or lunch; however, the granola may lose its crunch overnight, so it is best when eaten right away.

½ cup chopped fresh strawberries
¼ cup low-fat granola
1 8-ounce container plain low-fat yogurt

Place a third of the strawberries in the bottom of a parfait glass (or dish). Cover with half of the granola. Cover the granola with half the yogurt. Cover

YIELD: 1 serving

Nutritional Information Per Serving (1 parfait):
Calories: 241
Fat: 1.9 g
 Saturated Fat: 0.2 g
 Monounsaturated Fat: 0.4 g
 Polyunsaturated Fat: 1.2 g
Cholesterol: 5 mg
Sodium: 242 mg
Carbohydrate: 43.4 g
Dietary Fiber: 3.4 g
Sugars: 26.2 g
Starches: 13.7 g
Protein: 14.8 g
Diabetic Exchanges: 1½ Starch/Bread, ½ Fruit, 1 Fat-Free Milk

with half the remaining strawberries, then the remaining granola, then the remaining yogurt. Top with the rest of the strawberries. Serve immediately or refrigerate, covered, until ready to serve.

Soy Yogurt Smoothie

Soy milk is a creamy liquid derived from whole soybeans. It has a unique, somewhat nutty flavor and is an excellent source of protein, B vitamins, and iron. If you prefer, you can replace the soy milk with nonfat milk for an equally satisfying smoothie.

3 cups plain soy milk
1 small banana
1 teaspoon pure vanilla extract
1 cup strawberries
1 cup plain nonfat yogurt

Put all the ingredients into a blender and pulse for 10 to 20 seconds until well combined. Pour 1 cup into a glass and enjoy!

YIELD: 4 servings, 1 cup per serving

Nutritional Information Per Serving (1 cup):
Calories: 128
Fat: 3.8 g
  Saturated Fat: 0.4 g
  Monounsaturated Fat: 0.6 g
  Polyunsaturated Fat: 1.6 g
Cholesterol: 1 mg
Sodium: 70 mg
Carbohydrate: 16.4 g
Dietary Fiber: 3.8 g
Sugars: 4.4 g
Starches: 0 g
Protein: 8.8 g
Diabetic Exchanges: ½ Fruit, 1 Fat-Free Milk, ½ Fat

Hawaiian Sunrise

In addition to the contrasting colors, the different textures of the dried and fresh fruit in this low-fat dish make it interesting and refreshing for breakfast or lunch. It also holds up well for several hours in the refrigerator, so if you have a refrigerator at work, it makes an excellent bring-from-home lunch.

⅓ cup low-fat cottage cheese
1 tablespoon golden raisins
1 tablespoon dried cherries or cranberries
¼ cup unsweetened crushed pineapple
⅛ teaspoon ground cinnamon
½ 3-gram packet granulated fructose

Combine the cottage cheese, raisins, and cherries in a small bowl. Spread the pineapple out in a circle in the middle of a small plate. Spoon the cottage cheese mixture on top of the pineapple. Sprinkle with cinnamon and fructose and serve.

YIELD: 1 serving

Nutritional Information Per Serving:
Calories: 134
Fat: 0.9 g
  Saturated Fat: 0 g
  Monounsaturated Fat: 0.2 g
  Polyunsaturated Fat: 0 g
Cholesterol: 3 mg
Sodium: 294 mg
Carbohydrate: 23.8 g
Dietary Fiber: 1.4 g
Sugars: 7.2 g
Starches: 2.2 g
Protein: 10 g
Diabetic Exchanges: 1 Fruit, 1 Reduced-Fat Milk

Blueberry Blintzes Topped with Lime Crema

This tasty dish looks great, making it easy to impress your friends or family at breakfast or brunch. Make sure you seal the crepes to prevent the filling from leaking out. You can substitute fat-free or light ricotta cheese for the cottage cheese, if preferred.

For the Lime Crema:
¼ cup fat-free sour cream
2 teaspoons lime juice

For the Blintzes:
Canola cooking spray
¾ cup nonfat cottage cheese
¼ cup light cream cheese, softened
1 egg white
½ teaspoon grated lime zest
1 3-gram packet granulated fructose
¾ cup fresh blueberries, divided
6 7-inch crepes

YIELD: 6 servings, 1 blintz per serving

Nutritional Information Per Serving (1 blintz):
Calories: 180
Fat: 7.7 g
  Saturated Fat: 2.9 g
  Monounsaturated Fat: 2.9 g
  Polyunsaturated Fat: 1.3 g
Cholesterol: 88 mg
Sodium: 203 mg
Carbohydrate: 17.5 g
Dietary Fiber: 0.8 g
Sugars: 3.6 g
Starches: 1.6 g
Protein: 10 g
Diabetic Exchanges: 1 Fruit, 1 Reduced-Fat Milk

Preheat oven to 350 degrees F.

Prepare the lime crema by combining the sour cream with the lime juice in a small bowl. Refrigerate until ready to use.

Line a baking sheet with parchment paper or spray with cooking spray.

In a mixing bowl, combine the cottage cheese, cream cheese, egg white, lime zest, and fructose; blend until well combined. Stir in ½ cup blueberries.

Spoon ¼ cup cheese filling into the center of each crepe. Fold the top and bottom of the crepe over the filling and close the blintz by folding over the sides, forming a square pouch.

Place the stuffed blintzes on the prepared baking sheet, seam sides down. Bake for 10 to 12 minutes, or until filling is hot.

Serve each hot blintz topped with a dollop of chilled lime crema and a few fresh blueberries from the remaining ¼ cup.

Warm Scottish Oatmeal with Cranberries

This filling serving of Scottish oatmeal starts the day with a great source of dietary fiber. Studies have shown that including fiber in your diet may help reduce cholesterol levels. The fruit adds texture and sweetness, so you may not even want to add any pancake syrup.

½ cup Scottish oatmeal
1 tablespoon dried unsweetened cranberries
1 small banana, cut into ¼-inch slices
1 teaspoon sugar-free pancake syrup, optional

Prepare Scottish oatmeal according to package directions. While the oatmeal cooks, add the cranberries. Place the banana slices in a small bowl and top with the cooked oatmeal and cranberries. Drizzle with pancake syrup, if desired, and serve hot.

YIELD: 1 serving, ½ cup per serving

Nutritional Information Per Serving (½ cup):
Calories: 266
Fat: 3.6 g
  Saturated Fat: 0.7 g
  Monounsaturated Fat: 0.1 g
  Polyunsaturated Fat: 0.1 g
Cholesterol: 0 mg
Sodium: 1 mg
Carbohydrate: 56.6 g
Dietary Fiber: 7 g
Sugars: 12.4 g
Starches: 10.5 g
Protein: 7.1 g
Diabetic Exchanges:
  2 Starch/Bread, 2 Fruit

Cranberry Scones

These simple-to-make scones are great for breakfast or brunch. You can use dried cherries or raisins instead of dried cranberries if you prefer. You can also use orange zest instead of lemon zest. Enjoy with a hot cup of coffee or tea for a scrumptious treat.

Canola cooking spray
2½ cups all-purpose flour
4 teaspoons baking powder
½ teaspoon salt
¼ teaspoon baking soda
1 tablespoon granulated sugar
2 egg whites
3 tablespoons canola oil
1 cup low-fat buttermilk
½ cup dried cranberries
1 tablespoon grated lemon zest
1 egg white
½ teaspoon nonfat milk

Preheat oven to 400 degrees F.
  Lightly spray a large baking sheet with cooking spray.

YIELD: 12 scones, 1 scone per serving

Nutritional Information Per Serving (1 scone):
Calories: 159
Fat: 4.1 g
  Saturated Fat: 0.4 g
  Monounsaturated Fat: 1.5 g
  Polyunsaturated Fat: 1.7 g
Cholesterol: 1 mg
Sodium: 205 mg
Carbohydrate: 26.3 g
Dietary Fiber: 1.0 g
Sugars: 5.6 g
Starches: 0.5 g
Protein: 4.3 g
Diabetic Exchanges:
  1½ Starch/Bread, 1 Fat

In a large bowl, mix the flour, baking powder, salt, baking soda, and sugar.

In a small bowl, whisk together the 2 egg whites, oil, and buttermilk. Add to the flour mixture along with the dried cranberries and lemon zest, and mix with a fork until you have a sticky batter without any dry spots.

Spoon the scone batter onto the prepared baking sheet in 3½-inch by 2½-inch mounds, leaving at least 2 inches between the scones so they don't end up touching each other as they bake.

In a small bowl, whisk the egg white and milk. Using a pastry brush, lightly brush the top of each scone with the egg-white mixture.

Bake for 12 minutes, or until the tops of the scones are golden brown. Remove to a wire rack and allow to cool for a few minutes before serving. Once fully cooled each scone can be wrapped in plastic wrap and stored overnight in a cool place.

Cranberry Apple Muffins

These muffins are moist and flavorful. For something a little different, you can substitute dried blueberries, raisins, currants, dates, or cherries for the dried cranberries. Pack these in your family's lunches instead of junk food and processed snacks.

YIELD: 12 muffins, 1 muffin per serving

2 cups all-purpose flour
2 teaspoons baking powder
½ teaspoon baking soda
1 teaspoon ground cinnamon
1 3-gram packet granulated fructose
2 egg whites
2 tablespoons canola oil
½ cup apple cider
1 cup unsweetened applesauce
½ cup dried cranberries
⅓ cup diced apple (about 1 small apple)
Canola cooking spray

Preheat oven to 350 degrees F.

Mix all the ingredients, except cooking spray, in a large bowl until well combined.

Nutritional Information Per Serving (1 muffin):

Calories: 117
Fat: 2.7 g
  Saturated Fat: 0.3 g
  Monounsaturated Fat: 1.0 g
  Polyunsaturated Fat: 1.2 g
Cholesterol: 0 mg
Sodium: 71 mg
Carbohydrate: 20.5 g
Dietary Fiber: 1.2 g
Sugars: 2.5 g
Starches: 0.3 g
Protein: 2.8 g
Diabetic Exchanges:
  ½ Starch/Bread, 1 Fruit,
  ½ Fat

Lightly spray the cups of a muffin tin (standard 2½- by 1¼-inch size) with cooking spray. Pour the muffin batter into muffin tins and bake for 20 minutes, or until a toothpick inserted in the center comes out clean. Remove from oven and allow to cool a bit before handling and serving.

Cinnamon Buns

Cinnamon buns are one of the all-time great weekend breakfast treats. The raisins used in this version add a nice layer of sweetness, color, and texture. You can reheat leftover buns in the microwave on high for about 10 seconds, or until just hot (overheating will result in chewy buns).

1 teaspoon ground cinnamon
½ cup finely chopped golden raisins
½ tablespoon light margarine, melted
2 tablespoons pure honey
1 10-ounce can refrigerated low-fat buttermilk biscuits

Preheat oven to 400 degrees F.

In a small bowl, combine the cinnamon and raisins.

Cut a piece of parchment paper so it fits into the bottom of an 8-inch round cake pan and comes up the sides at least an inch.

Brush the parchment paper with the margarine and sprinkle the cinnamon and raisin mixture evenly over it. Drizzle the honey over the cinnamon and raisin layer. Arrange the biscuits in one layer, touching each other, on top of the raisin mixture.

Bake 10 to 12 minutes, or until the tops of the biscuits are golden brown. Run a rubber spatula around the edge of the pan to loosen any biscuits that may be attached to the sides.

Place a serving plate on top of the pan of biscuits. Pick up both the pan and the plate and flip over, inverting the biscuits onto the plate. Slide the pan and parchment paper off to reveal your warm cinnamon buns (tap once or twice if they stick to the pan).

YIELD: 10 buns, 1 bun per serving

Nutritional Information Per Serving (1 bun):

Calories: 88
Fat: 1.1 g
 Saturated Fat: 0.1 g
 Monounsaturated Fat: 0.1 g
 Polyunsaturated Fat: 0.1 g
Cholesterol: 0 mg
Sodium: 185 mg
Carbohydrate: 19.4 g
Dietary Fiber: 0.9 g
Sugars: 9.2 g
Starches: 1.2 g
Protein: 1.8 g
Diabetic Exchanges:
 1½ Starch/Bread

6

Appetizers, Soups, and Salads

Shrimp Diane

Warm Spinach-Artichoke Dip

Sweet Onion Dip

Mexican Black Bean and Cheese Dip

Tuna Pâté

Salmon Cakes

Grilled Chicken Quesadilla

Spinach Bruschetta

Garlic Crostini

Potato Skins

Tandoori Chicken Skewers

Baked Onion Rings

Buffalo-Style Chicken Thumbs

Homemade Chicken Broth

Homemade Beef Broth

Homemade Vegetable Broth

French Onion Soup

Gazpacho for Four

Hearty Chicken Vegetable Soup

Sausage Cannellini Soup

Hot and Sour Soup

Corn and Crabmeat Chowder

Cream of Broccoli Soup

Sherried Cream of Carrot Soup

Pasta e Fagiole Soup

Brazilian Smoked Black Bean Soup

Tortellini Soup with Escarole

Carrot Salad

Corn and Black Bean Salad

Greek Salad

Mediterranean Bean and Tuna Salad

Refreshing Spring Tabbouleh

Lemon-Garlic Salad

Soho Sirloin Salad

Sicilian Salad

House Salad

Caprese Salad

Busy Tuna Salad

Balsamic Chicken Salad

Big Cobb Salad

Asian Cabbage Salad

Creamy Coleslaw

Appetizers can provide a nice start to a meal, whetting the appetite for what is to come. Ranging from simple finger foods and colorful salads to dips and pâté, they are also standard fare when you are entertaining guests,

Many of the appetizers served in restaurants have enough calories, fat, and cholesterol to meet a full day's allowance, with fried dishes such as Buffalo-style chicken wings and battered, fried whole onions topping the list. Then, of course, there's the dip or sauce that comes with them! Most people realize that a majority of restaurant food is made to taste good regardless of the health consequences, but how many people would guess that a fried onion could contain 60 grams of fat?

We've included several modified versions of the most notorious restaurant favorites for you to nosh on without breaking the nutritional bank. In the mood for something deep-fried? Try our Baked Onion Rings with a side of Zesty Dipping Sauce, Potato Skins, or Buffalo-Style Chicken Thumbs. How about something to dip into? Try our Warm Spinach-Artichoke Dip or Mexican Black Bean and Cheese Dip. Having some friends over? Dish out some Spinach Bruschetta, Garlic Crostini, or Salmon Cakes. All of these appetizers are delicious alternatives to their restaurant counterparts and are significantly healthier.

The term "salad" refers not only to the small tossed lettuce salads that often start off a meal, such as our House Salad, but it essentially includes any food or mixture of foods that get tossed with, or accompanied or topped by, a dressing. Salads can include main dishes such as Balsamic Chicken Salad, in which a marinated, grilled chicken breast is set on top of a bed of lettuce tossed with carrots, tomato, and balsamic vinegar. Salads are also associated with picnics or served as accompaniments, such as Creamy Coleslaw or Corn and Black Bean Salad.

Tossed salads are incredibly versatile. They can be served as main dishes, side dishes, or appetizers. Salads can be a wonderful addition to a meal, especially if you find that you are still hungry after a meal, or if you find yourself reaching for second helpings. Smaller tossed salads, like our House Salad, provide a great way to puff up a meal without adding enough calories and carbohydrate to throw off your meal plan. Still hungry after eating properly portioned meals? Add another cup or two of lettuce to your tossed salad. One cup of lettuce contains only about 5 calories and less than 1 gram of carbohydrate, and it is much better than eating another piece of chicken or a second helping of pasta.

Unfortunately, the healthful benefits offered by salads are often outweighed by the "accessories" added to them. Adding fattening cheese or deli meats and high-fat dressings and sauces can turn a nutritionally sound salad into something quite the opposite. It's hard to believe, but sometimes ordering a salad with regular dressing in a restaurant is worse than ordering a burger or steak!

The English word "soup" is derived from the word "sop," which referred to a dish consisting of bread topped with roast juices. Soup has come a long way since then, with various types and styles that include cream soups, thin soups, thick soups, broths, chowders, bisques, and chilled soups. A soup can contain just about anything, from fresh ingredients to leftovers, provided it starts off with a good base. We have included recipes for Homemade Chicken Broth, Homemade Beef Broth, and Homemade Vegetable Broth. All three are good bases for soups, sauces, and other dishes, and are also low in calories, sodium, and fat. We highly suggest that you make your own broth for using in recipes and store it in small batches in the freezer. If you must use canned broth, you can reduce the sodium content by adding ⅔ cup water to each 1 cup of broth.

Soup can be served as an appetizer, a side dish, or a main dish. For example, our Pasta e Fagiole Soup is a meal within itself, while our chilled Gazpacho for Four is better served as a light lunch or as an appetizer. Last, soups are good any time of the year. Don't wait until the dead of winter before you think about eating soup. Spring and summer are great times for soup, especially since farmers' markets are overflowing with fresh fruits and vegetables. A soup that is traditionally served hot can be served at room temperature and enjoyed even in the dog days of summer.

Shrimp Diane

Shrimp and mushrooms are tossed with a spicy wine sauce and served with a slice of crisp Italian bread. This recipe doubles easily and makes a great dish for a larger dinner party when served with Garlic Crostini (page 61) instead of the simpler Italian bread.

1 teaspoon canola oil
1 teaspoon margarine
2 tablespoons minced shallots
1 cup thinly sliced white mushrooms
16 jumbo shrimp, peeled and deveined (about 1 pound)
¼ cup dry white wine
½ teaspoon ground cayenne pepper
⅛ teaspoon freshly ground black pepper
Pinch salt substitute
2 tablespoons sliced scallions
1 tablespoon cream sherry
4 ½-inch-thick slices Italian bread
Canola or olive oil cooking spray
2 tablespoons chopped fresh parsley

YIELD: 4 servings, can be doubled

Nutritional Information Per Serving (¼ of recipe):

Calories: 167
Fat: 3.9 g
  Saturated Fat: 0.3 g
  Monounsaturated Fat: 1.2 g
  Polyunsaturated Fat: 1.5 g
Cholesterol: 134 mg
Sodium: 206 mg
Carbohydrate: 8.2 g
Dietary Fiber: 0.7 g
Sugars: 0.6 g
Starches: 4.8 g
Protein: 19.5 g
Diabetic Exchanges:
  1 Starch/Bread, 1 Medium-Fat Meat

Preheat oven to 400 degrees F.

In a large nonstick skillet, heat the oil and margarine over medium heat until the margarine melts. Add the shallots and sauté for 1 minute. Add the mushrooms and sauté until they become tender. Add the shrimp, wine, cayenne pepper, black pepper, salt substitute, scallions, and sherry. Cover and cook, stirring occasionally, until the shrimp become pink and firm to touch, about 5 minutes.

Meanwhile, arrange the bread slices on a baking sheet and spray lightly with cooking spray; bake until just crisp.

Stir half the parsley into the shrimp, then divide equally among 4 dinner plates. Sprinkle with the remaining parsley and serve with a slice of warm bread on the side of the plate.

Warm Spinach-Artichoke Dip

This warm dip is similar to those served in restaurant chains, but it's low in fat and has a fraction of the calories and sodium. It's virtually guilt-free and is perfect for parties and get-togethers. Serve with pita wedges, baked tortilla chips, or low-fat crackers.

YIELD: 12 servings,
2 tablespoons per serving

Nutritional Information
Per Serving
(2 tablespoons):

Calories: 71
Fat: 2.5 g
  Saturated Fat: 1.2 g
  Monounsaturated Fat: 0.8 g
  Polyunsaturated Fat: 0.2 g
Cholesterol: 7 mg
Sodium: 196 mg
Carbohydrate: 6.5 g
Dietary Fiber: 2.2 g
Sugars: 1.4 g
Starches: 0.9 g
Protein: 7.3 g
Diabetic Exchanges:
  2 Vegetable, ½ Fat

Canola cooking spray
1 teaspoon olive oil
2 tablespoon minced onion
1 small clove garlic, minced
½ cup light sour cream
1½ cups low-fat cottage cheese
2 egg whites
1 tablespoon grated Parmesan cheese
2 teaspoons fresh lemon juice
½ teaspoon hot pepper sauce
Pinch white pepper
⅛ teaspoon crushed red pepper flakes
2 10-ounce packages frozen chopped spinach,
  thawed and squeezed dry
1 10-ounce package frozen artichoke hearts,
  thawed, patted dry, and halved
2 tablespoons chopped roasted red pepper
2 tablespoons shredded reduced-fat Monterey Jack
  cheese
⅓ cup thinly sliced scallions, green part only

Preheat oven to 350 degrees F. Lightly coat a 1½-quart casserole with cooking spray.

Heat a small nonstick skillet over medium heat. Away from the heat source, spray with cooking spray, and return to the heat. Add the oil and onion and sauté until softened, about 5 minutes. Stir in the garlic and sauté for another minute; set aside.

In a food processor, process the sour cream, cottage cheese, egg whites, Parmesan cheese, lemon juice, hot sauce, white pepper, and red pepper flakes until smooth.

In a large mixing bowl, combine the spinach, artichoke hearts, roasted red pepper, Monterey

Jack cheese, and the cottage cheese mixture. Spoon evenly into the casserole, cover, and bake for 25 minutes, or until the center of the dip is hot. Sprinkle with scallions and serve hot.

Sweet Onion Dip

For this dish, you'll find that the sweeter the onion, the better the dip will be. We used Vidalia onions, but most varieties of yellow onion work well as long as you sauté them long enough. Not only is this easy to make and delicious, it is also low in calories, fat, sodium, cholesterol, and carbohydrate. Serve with pita wedges or cut fresh vegetables.

YIELD: 16 servings, 2 tablespoons per serving

Canola cooking spray
1 teaspoon canola oil
1 teaspoon light margarine
1 small Vidalia onion, finely chopped
2 cups plain low-fat yogurt
½ teaspoon white vinegar
1 tablespoon minced fresh parsley
¼ teaspoon salt substitute
¼ teaspoon black pepper, or to taste

Nutritional Information Per Serving (2 tablespoons):

Calories: 24
Fat: 0.9 g
  Saturated Fat: 0.4 g
  Monounsaturated Fat: 0.3 g
  Polyunsaturated Fat: 0.2 g
Cholesterol: 2 mg
Sodium: 23 mg
Carbohydrate: 2.6 g
Dietary Fiber: 0.1 g
Sugars: 2.1 g
Starches: 0 g
Protein: 1.7 g
Diabetic Exchanges:
  1 Vegetable

Heat a nonstick skillet over medium-low heat. Away from the heat source, spray with cooking spray and return to the heat. Add the canola oil and margarine. Add the onions and sauté until very soft and golden brown, about 15 to 20 minutes.

Transfer the onions to a large bowl and combine with the yogurt, vinegar, parsley, salt substitute, and pepper. Serve while slightly warm or cover and refrigerate until chilled.

Mexican Black Bean and Cheese Dip

This dip is good with baked tortilla chips or whole wheat pita wedges. You can also use it to top baked nachos or as a filling for tacos and burritos. If you prefer a chunkier dip, skip the step that calls for the food processor.

YIELD: 14 servings, ¼ cup per serving

1 cup chopped yellow onion
1 tablespoon canola oil
1 large clove garlic, minced
4 15.5-ounce cans low-sodium black beans, rinsed and drained
1 cup water
3 ounces fat-free cream cheese (about ⅓ of an 8-ounce package)
⅓ cup shredded mild or sharp reduced-fat, reduced-sodium Cheddar cheese
2 tablespoons sliced scallions, green part only
2 tablespoons pickled jalapeño pepper slices, optional

Nutritional Information Per Serving (¼ cup):

Calories: 138
Fat: 1.7 g
  Saturated Fat: 0.2 g
  Monounsaturated Fat: 0.5 g
  Polyunsaturated Fat: 0.7 g
Cholesterol: 2 mg
Sodium: 153 mg
Carbohydrate: 21.8 g
Dietary Fiber: 7.7 g
Sugars: 2.2 g
Starches: 11.1 g
Protein: 9.5 g
Diabetic Exchanges:
  1 Starch/Bread, 1 Very Lean Meat, 1 Vegetable

In a medium saucepan, sauté the onion in the canola oil over medium heat until soft. Add the garlic and sauté for another minute, stirring often. Add the beans and water; stir until well mixed. Reduce heat to low, cover, and simmer for 30 minutes, stirring occasionally (if the water cooks off, add more, 2 tablespoons at a time, to prevent the beans from burning). Stir in ⅓ cup water, and mix with a wooden spoon so the beans break apart and the mixture becomes creamy.

Preheat oven to 375 degrees F.

Spoon the bean mixture into a food processor and process for 30 seconds, or until smooth.

Spoon ⅓ of the bean mixture into an 8-inch round casserole that is at least 3 inches high and spread evenly. (This is a great dish to serve on a buffet, so you can also prepare it in a chafing dish and serve in a steam table.) Scatter bits of the cream cheese on top of the bean layer. Spoon the remaining bean mixture over the cream cheese layer and spread evenly so that all of the cream cheese is covered. Sprinkle with the Cheddar cheese and bake for 20 minutes.

Remove from the oven and sprinkle with scallions and jalapeño pepper slices, if desired. Place the casserole on a heat-safe trivet and serve from the baking dish.

Tuna Pâté

Relatively simple to prepare and nutritionally low on the guilt scale, this pâté is perfect for a party or get-together and can be doubled. You can also use it for canapés by spooning 1-tablespoon portions on bread crisps and garnishing with parsley sprigs.

1 cup low-fat cottage cheese
2 tablespoons chopped scallions, green parts only
4 teaspoons minced fresh parsley, divided
½ teaspoon dried dill
1½ teaspoons reduced-sodium soy sauce
½ teaspoon Worcestershire sauce
⅛ teaspoon freshly ground black pepper
1 7-ounce can water-packed white albacore tuna, drained
parsley sprigs, optional garnish
lemon wedges, optional garnish
Italian bread, thinly sliced and toasted in the oven, or low-fat crackers, or pita wedges, optional

In a food processor, purée the cottage cheese. Add the scallions, 1 teaspoon parsley, dill, soy sauce, Worcestershire sauce, pepper, and tuna. Process until just smooth.

Line a small pâté or loaf pan with plastic wrap. Scatter 1 tablespoon parsley on the bottom of the pan. (You can use individual ramekins or a regular bowl if that's what you have on hand.) Spoon the tuna mixture into the pan and push down to pack firmly. Refrigerate overnight.

To serve, invert onto a serving plate and garnish with parsley sprigs and lemon wedges, if desired. Serve with toasted Italian bread slices, low-fat crackers, or pita wedges.

YIELD: 16 servings, 2 tablespoons per serving

Nutritional Information Per Serving (2 tablespoons):
Calories: 22
Fat: 0.3 g
  Saturated Fat: 0 g
  Monounsaturated Fat: 0 g
  Polyunsaturated Fat: 0 g
Cholesterol: 1 mg
Sodium: 74 mg
Carbohydrate: 0.8 g
Dietary Fiber: 0 g
Sugars: 0.5 g
Starches: 0.1 g
Protein: 4.1 g
Diabetic Exchanges: 1 Very Lean Meat

Salmon Cakes

Canned salmon works very well for this dish, but it does add to the overall sodium content. You can always poach fresh salmon and chill it before using in this recipe in place of the canned salmon. You can also shape the salmon mixture into 3½-ounce patties, broil, and serve on burger buns with lettuce, onion, and tomato. Leftover cakes can be reheated in a toaster oven or microwave until heated through.

YIELD: 7 servings, 2 cakes per serving

Nutritional Information Per Serving (2 cakes):

Calories: 169
Fat: 5.9 g
  Saturated Fat: 1.3 g
  Monounsaturated Fat: 2.2 g
  Polyunsaturated Fat: 1.6 g
Cholesterol: 55 mg
Sodium: 304 mg
Carbohydrate: 12.2 g
Dietary Fiber: 0.5 g
Sugars: 0.6 g
Starches: 0.2 g
Protein: 15.9 g
Diabetic Exchanges:
  1 Starch/Bread, 1 Medium-
  Fat Meat

1 14-ounce can low-sodium salmon, drained
1 egg
2 egg whites
2 tablespoons Dijon mustard
1 cup unseasoned bread crumbs
1½ teaspoons hot pepper sauce
1 teaspoon lemon juice
1 shallot, minced
1 teaspoon dried parsley flakes
⅛ teaspoon black pepper
Canola cooking spray
lemon wedges

Combine all the ingredients in a bowl and form into 14 patties.

Conventional oven method: Line a baking sheet with aluminum foil and spray lightly with cooking spray. Place the patties on the baking sheet and spray lightly with cooking spray. Broil about 8 inches from the heat source for 4 minutes, then flip and broil for another 4 minutes, or until golden brown and heated through.

Toaster oven method: Line the toaster oven tray with aluminum foil and spray lightly with cooking spray. Arrange the patties on the tray, fitting as many as possible in one layer. Spray the patties lightly with cooking spray. Broil for 4 or 5 minutes, flip, then broil for another 3 or 4 minutes, or until golden brown and heated through.

Serve with lemon wedges and a dip, such as Cajun Tartar Sauce (page 208), Zesty Dipping Sauce (page 211), Simple Sour Cream and Dijon Dip (page 212), or Creamy Creole Dip (page 212).

Grilled Chicken Quesadilla

This recipe can be modified to accommodate different fillings, so feel free to improvise and have fun with it. Try grilled vegetables or lean beef, rice and beans. If you have any leftover chicken from making Homemade Chicken Broth (page 66), that will also work well.

YIELD: 6 servings,
3 wedges per serving

Nutritional Information Per Serving (3 wedges):

Calories: 200
Fat: 5.3 g
  Saturated Fat: 1.7 g
  Monounsaturated Fat: 0.8 g
  Polyunsaturated Fat: 0.2 g
Cholesterol: 16 mg
Sodium: 340 mg
Carbohydrate: 20.8 g
Dietary Fiber: 1.7 g
Sugars: 1.9 g
Starches: 0.1 g
Protein: 16.1 g
Diabetic Exchanges:
  1½ Starch/Bread, 2 Very
  Lean Meat, ½ Fat

Canola cooking spray
1 3-ounce piece boneless, skinless chicken breast, pounded to ¼-inch thick
4 8-inch reduced-fat whole wheat flour tortillas
1 cup shredded reduced-fat, reduced-sodium, sharp Cheddar cheese
¼ cup seeded chopped tomato
¼ cup chopped roasted red pepper
¼ cup sliced scallions, green part only
2 tablespoons chopped jalapeño pepper slices, optional
Nonfat or light sour cream, optional
Fat-Free Salsa (page 213), or store-bought fat-free salsa, optional

Preheat oven to 375 degrees F.

Heat a grill pan over medium heat until hot. Away from the heat source, spray lightly with cooking spray and return to the heat. If using an outdoor grill, heat to medium heat. Grill the chicken breast until cooked through. Cut the chicken into thin bite-size pieces.

Lay 2 tortillas on a large nonstick baking sheet and sprinkle each with ½ cup shredded cheese. Divide the sliced chicken, chopped tomato, red pepper, scallions, and jalapeño pepper, if desired, among the tortillas, scattering evenly over the cheese.

Place the remaining tortillas over each filled tortilla so the edges meet; press down firmly. Bake for 5 minutes, or until the cheese melts.

Using a sharp knife, cut each quesadilla into 6 wedges. Serve hot with nonfat sour cream and salsa, if desired.

Spinach Bruschetta

Sliced Italian bread is toasted until golden and topped with fresh spinach and seasoned tomatoes. Refreshing, easy to make, and visually stimulating, Spinach Bruschetta are also a great way to use up day-old bread. This recipe can easily be doubled, and the tomato topping can be kept, covered and refrigerated, overnight. Squeeze a bit of fresh lemon over each slice before serving, if desired.

**YIELD: 6 servings,
2 bruschetta per serving**

**Nutritional Information
Per Serving (2 bruschetta):**

Calories: 43
Fat: 0.6 g
  Saturated Fat: 0.1 g
  Monounsaturated Fat: 0.1 g
  Polyunsaturated Fat: 0.2 g
Cholesterol: 0 mg
Sodium: 68 mg
Carbohydrate: 8.4 g
Dietary Fiber: 1.1 g
Sugars: 0.3 g
Starches: 4.9 g
Protein: 1.6 g
Diabetic Exchanges:
  2 Vegetable

3 large Roma or plum tomatoes, seeded and
　　chopped (about 2 cups)
2 tablespoons chopped fresh basil
2 cloves garlic, minced
1 teaspoon lemon juice
Pinch salt
Dash ground black pepper, or to taste
5 ounces fresh spinach, cleaned, stems removed
　　(½ of a 10-ounce bag commonly found in super-
　　markets)
12 ¼-inch-thick slices Italian bread, about ½ small
　　loaf (Don't buy a huge loaf of bread. Choose a
　　loaf that is only about 3 or 4 inches wide. The
　　¼-inch-thick slices of bread should be about
　　3 inches long by 2 inches wide.)
Olive oil cooking spray
Several lemon wedges, for garnish

In a medium bowl, mix the tomatoes, basil, garlic, lemon juice, salt, and black pepper. Cover and refrigerate until chilled, about 2 hours.

Preheat oven to 400 degrees F.

Place the spinach in a large microwave-safe bowl. Cover with a microwave-safe plate and heat for 30 seconds, or until spinach leaves wilt slightly. Remove the spinach to a clean towel and pat dry; set aside.

Place the bread slices on a nonstick baking sheet. Lightly spray the top of the bread slices with cooking spray. Bake for about 10 minutes, or until the bread becomes crisp and golden around the edges.

Arrange the toasted bread on a large platter. Divide the spinach leaves among the slices of toasted bread. Top the spinach with 2 tablespoons chilled tomato mixture, leaving behind the additional liquid. Garnish with lemon wedges and serve at once.

Garlic Crostini

This is an excellent alternative to typical garlic bread, which is usually loaded with butter and thickly sliced, and is also a great way to use day-old or stale bread. Garlic Crostini are crisp, full of flavor, and make a perfect accompaniment to soups, salads, and main entrées. Serve it with our Soho Sirloin Salad (page 85), Gazpacho for Four (page 70), or Classic Italian Meatballs in Pomodoro Sauce (page 132).

YIELD: 4 servings, 2 slices per serving

Nutritional Information Per Serving (2 slices):

Calories: 66
Fat: 1.8 g
　Saturated Fat: 0.3 g
　Monounsaturated Fat: 1 g
　Polyunsaturated Fat: 0.4 g
Cholesterol: 0 mg
Sodium: 117 mg
Carbohydrate: 10.4 g
Dietary Fiber: 0.6 g
Sugars: 0.2 g
Starches: 9.7 g
Protein: 1.8 g
Diabetic Exchanges:
　½ Starch/Bread, ½ Fat

1 teaspoon olive oil
¼ teaspoon no-salt Italian seasoning
1 large garlic clove, finely minced (about 1 tablespoon)
2 tablespoons minced fresh parsley, or 1 teaspoon dried parsley flakes
Pinch ground black pepper
8 ¼-inch-thick slices Italian bread, about ½ small loaf (Don't buy a huge loaf of bread. Choose a loaf that is only about 3 or 4 inches wide. The ¼-inch-thick slices of bread should be about 3 inches long by 2 inches wide.)
Canola or olive oil cooking spray

Preheat oven to 400 degrees F.

In a small bowl, mix the olive oil, Italian seasoning, garlic, parsley, and black pepper.

Place the bread slices on a nonstick baking sheet. Spread the garlic mixture on the bread. Lightly spray the top of the bread slices with cooking spray. Bake for 7 to 10 minutes, or until the bread becomes crisp and golden around the edges and the garlic becomes golden.

Arrange the toasted bread on a large platter and serve.

Potato Skins

This version of the popular restaurant and tavern appetizer is much healthier but every bit as satisfying. These are best when you bake the potatoes the night before and refrigerate them overnight, but you can bake them the same day if necessary.

4 large russet potatoes, scrubbed, baked, refrigerated overnight or until cold
1 teaspoon salt substitute
½ teaspoon ground black pepper
Canola cooking spray
2 slices turkey bacon, cooked crisp and finely chopped
1 cup shredded reduced-fat, reduced-sodium Cheddar cheese
4 tablespoons fat-free sour cream
¼ cup thinly sliced scallions, green part only

Slice the cooked potatoes in half lengthwise and scoop out enough of the potato flesh to leave about ¼ inch on the skin; discard the scooped-out potato flesh. Cut each potato into thirds, crosswise, and season lightly with salt substitute and black pepper.

Line a baking sheet with aluminum foil and spray with cooking spray. Arrange the potato skins on the baking sheet and spray with cooking spray until lightly coated.

Broil the potato skins for 3 to 5 minutes, or until they are crisp and golden brown. Remove from the oven and top with chopped turkey bacon and shredded cheese. Return to the oven and broil until cheese melts, about 1 minute.

For each serving, top 3 potato pieces with 1 tablespoon sour cream sprinkled with sliced scallions.

YIELD: 8 servings, 3 pieces per serving

Nutritional Information Per Serving (3 pieces):

Calories: 121
Fat: 2.7 g
  Saturated Fat: 1.2 g
  Monounsaturated Fat: 0.7 g
  Polyunsaturated Fat: 0.2 g
Cholesterol: 9 mg
Sodium: 231 mg
Carbohydrate: 15.4 g
Dietary Fiber: 2.4 g
Sugars: 1.3 g
Starches: 11 g
Protein: 8.9 g
Diabetic Exchanges:
  ½ Starch/Bread,
  ½ Reduced-Fat Milk

Tandoori Chicken Skewers

This sensational party appetizer can be easily doubled. You can also make this into a dinner entrée for four by serving the skewers with couscous or brown rice and some grilled vegetables. Soak wooden skewers in water for about 30 minutes before using to help prevent them from burning in the oven or on the grill.

½ cup low-fat plain yogurt
2 cloves garlic, minced
¾ teaspoon ground cumin
Pinch ground cloves
1 tablespoon grated fresh ginger
¼ teaspoon chili powder
⅛ teaspoon paprika
1 teaspoon lemon juice
¼ teaspoon salt substitute
1 pound boneless, skinless chicken breasts
Canola cooking spray
Lemon or lime wedges, optional

YIELD: 14 servings, 2 skewers per serving

Nutritional Information Per Serving (2 skewers):

Calories: 61
Fat: 1.3 g
  Saturated Fat: 0.4 g
  Monounsaturated Fat: 0.5 g
  Polyunsaturated Fat: 0.2 g
Cholesterol: 28 mg
Sodium: 31 mg
Carbohydrate: 0.9 g
Dietary Fiber: 0.1 g
Sugars: 0.8 g
Starches: 0 g
Protein: 10.6 g
Diabetic Exchanges: 1 Very
  Lean Meat, ½ Fat

In a bowl, combine the yogurt, garlic, cumin, cloves, ginger, chili powder, paprika, lemon juice, and salt substitute.

Pound the chicken so it is no thicker than ½ inch. Cut the chicken into ¼-inch slices and place in a large resealable plastic bag along with the marinade. Shift the chicken around in the bag to coat it well with the marinade and refrigerate several hours, preferably overnight.

Preheat oven to 425 degrees F (or heat an outdoor grill to medium).

If using the oven, spray a roasting pan with cooking spray. Thread the marinated chicken slices on 7-inch wooden skewers, one piece of chicken per skewer; discard remaining marinade. Arrange the skewered chicken on the roasting pan and bake until cooked through, about 7 minutes. If grilling, grill for 3 or 4 minutes per side, or until cooked through. Serve with lemon or lime wedges, if desired.

Baked Onion Rings

These baked onion rings are better than a lot of the deep-fried onion rings in restaurants, with only a fraction of the fat, calories, cholesterol, and sodium. Now how can you argue with that? Try these with our Zesty Dipping Sauce (page 211) for a real treat.

Canola cooking spray
8 low-salt snack crackers, such as Ritz, crushed
¼ cup unseasoned bread crumbs
2 tablespoons all-purpose flour
½ teaspoon paprika
¼ teaspoon garlic powder
¼ teaspoon salt substitute
5 egg whites
2 teaspoons evaporated nonfat milk
2 Vidalia onions, sliced into ½-inch-thick rings

Preheat oven to 375 degrees F.

Line a baking sheet with aluminum foil and spray with cooking spray.

In a medium bowl, combine the crushed crackers, bread crumbs, flour, paprika, garlic powder, and salt substitute.

In a separate bowl, whisk the egg whites and milk until frothy.

Discard the smaller onion rings or save for another use. You should be left with between 6 and 8 onion ring slices.

Dip 1 slice of onion first in the egg mixture, then into the crumb mixture, coating the onion lightly with the crumb mixture. Return the lightly coated onion to the egg mixture and then back to the crumb mixture for a final coating. Continue until all the rings are breaded, arranging the breaded rings on the baking sheet in a single layer. Note that you will not need to use all of the egg mixture or crumb mixture, so discard what is left over.

Spray the top of the onion rings lightly with cooking spray, flip, and lightly spray the other side. Bake for 15 minutes, or until golden and crisp. Serve hot.

YIELD: 2 servings, can be doubled

**Nutritional Information
Per Serving (½ of recipe):**

Calories: 167
Fat: 2.9 g
  Saturated Fat: 0.5 g
  Monounsaturated Fat: 1.2 g
  Polyunsaturated Fat: 1 g
Cholesterol: 0 mg
Sodium: 250 mg
Carbohydrate: 25 g
Dietary Fiber: 1.7 g
Sugars: 2 g
Starches: 0.4 g
Protein: 9.9 g
Diabetic Exchanges:
  1 Starch/Bread, 2 Vegetable, 1 Fat

Buffalo-Style Chicken Thumbs

Hot and spicy chicken wings without all the fat and calories—or those pesky chicken bones! Serve with some low-fat or fat-free blue cheese dressing and celery sticks and you're all set for a football game.

YIELD: 4 servings

**Nutritional Information
Per Serving (¼ of recipe):**
Calories: 149
Fat: 2.6 g
  Saturated Fat: 0.6 g
  Monounsaturated Fat: 0.8 g
  Polyunsaturated Fat: 0.7 g
Cholesterol: 48 mg
Sodium: 145 mg
Carbohydrate: 8.1 g
Dietary Fiber: 0.3 g
Sugars: 0.1 g
Starches: 0 g
Protein: 22.1 g
Diabetic Exchanges:
  ½ Starch/Bread, 3 Very Lean
  Meat

Canola cooking spray
3 egg whites
1 pound boneless, skinless chicken breast, fat-
  trimmed, cut into bite-size pieces
¼ cup all-purpose flour
Pinch ground black pepper
½ cup unseasoned bread crumbs
2 teaspoons light margarine
⅔ cup hot pepper sauce
Fat-free blue cheese dressing, optional
Celery sticks, optional

Preheat oven to 375 degrees F.

Line a baking sheet with aluminum foil and spray with cooking spray.

Whisk the egg whites in a medium bowl until frothy. Add the chicken pieces and stir to coat.

Combine the flour, pepper, and bread crumbs in another medium bowl.

Using a fork, place 1 egg-coated chicken piece into the crumb mixture; lightly coat and place on the baking sheet. Repeat with remaining pieces of chicken.

Bake the chicken for 15 minutes, or until it is cooked through.

Meanwhile, heat the margarine and hot sauce in a small saucepan over medium heat, stirring, until it simmers for 1 minute. Cover and set aside.

Remove the cooked chicken to a mixing bowl and toss with the warm hot sauce until well coated. Serve at once with fat-free blue cheese dressing and celery sticks, if desired.

Homemade Chicken Broth

Making healthy, delicious homemade broth is so simple that it's a shame more people don't do it. While there are good reduced-sodium, low-fat store-bought broths available, nothing beats the real thing. Store in several different size freezer-safe containers until ready to use. Use the chicken meat instead of grilled chicken in Grilled Chicken Quesadilla (page 59) or in Hearty White Chili (page 100). You can keep the chicken in the freezer in a resealable freezer bag for about a month.

YIELD: About 14 cups broth, plus about 5 cups chicken meat

Nutritional Information Per Serving (1 cup):

Calories: 20
Fat: 0.6 g
  Saturated Fat: 0.2 g
  Monounsaturated Fat: 0.2 g
  Polyunsaturated Fat: 0.2 g
Cholesterol: 2 mg
Sodium: 20 mg
Carbohydrate: 3 g
Dietary Fiber: 0.8 g
Sugars: 0.2 g
Starches: 0 g
Protein: 1 g
Diabetic Exchanges: Free

3 large carrots, peeled and quartered
2 stalks celery, quartered
1 large yellow onion, quartered
6 sprigs fresh parsley
3 cloves garlic, peeled and halved
½ teaspoon dried thyme
1 teaspoon whole black peppercorns
1 bay leaf
1 5-pound whole chicken, gizzard and liver
  discarded
4 quarts water, approximately

Place all the ingredients in a large stockpot, making sure the water covers everything—including the chicken. Bring to a boil over high heat. Reduce heat and simmer for 2½ hours, skimming off and discarding the foam that rises to the top every 20 minutes, or as needed.

Strain the broth through a colander or China cap into a second stockpot or saucepan. Set the cooked chicken aside and discard the remaining solids. Refrigerate the broth overnight.

Once the chicken is cool enough to handle, pick the chicken meat off the bones and refrigerate or freeze for later use.

The fat remaining in the broth will solidify at the top overnight. Skim off the layer of fat using a spoon or rubber spatula and discard. Use the defatted broth immediately or freeze in various size containers for later use (we suggest sizes ranging from 1 to 4 cups).

Homemade Beef Broth

This beef broth is not only low-sodium and low-fat, it is also flavorful and delicious. Take the time to make your own broth and freeze it in several different size containers until you need it. You can use this broth for French Onion Soup (page 69).

Canola cooking spray
3 pounds beef shanks
10 cups water
4 celery stalks, cut into quarters
2 medium carrots, peeled and cut into thirds
1 large onion, quartered
3 cloves garlic, peeled and halved
1 bay leaf
10 whole black peppercorns
3 sprigs fresh parsley

Heat a large stockpot over medium-high heat. Spray with cooking spray and cook the beef shanks until browned, turning often, about 12 minutes.

Add the water and remaining ingredients and bring to a boil. Cover, reduce heat, and simmer over low heat for 2 hours.

Strain the broth into a second stockpot. Discard the solids. Cover and refrigerate the strained broth overnight.

Much of the fat remaining in the broth will solidify at the top overnight. Skim off the layer of fat using a spoon or rubber spatula and discard. Use the defatted broth immediately or freeze in various size containers for later use (we suggest sizes ranging from 1 to 4 cups).

YIELD: About 8 cups, or 16 ($\frac{1}{2}$ cup) servings

Nutritional Information Per Serving ($\frac{1}{2}$ cup):

Calories: 16
Fat: 0.4 g
  Saturated Fat: 0.1 g
  Monounsaturated Fat: 0.2 g
  Polyunsaturated Fat: 0 g
Cholesterol: 4 mg
Sodium: 15 mg
Carbohydrate: 1.2 g
Dietary Fiber: 0.3 g
Sugars: 0.1 g
Starches: 0.1 g
Protein: 2.0 g
Diabetic Exchanges: Free

Homemade Vegetable Broth

This flavorful vegetable broth can be used in place of chicken broth in many recipes. You can also use it to cook couscous, vegetables, rice—any number of foods. It is easy to make and infinitely better than what you would get in a store because it isn't loaded with salt and fat. Store the broth in several different size freezer-safe containers until ready to use.

YIELD: About 8 cups, or 16 (½ cup) servings

Nutritional Information Per Serving (½ cup):

Calories: 13
Fat: 0.2 g
  Saturated Fat: 0 g
  Monounsaturated Fat: 0.1 g
  Polyunsaturated Fat: 0.1 g
Cholesterol: 0 mg
Sodium: 15 mg
Carbohydrate: 2.8 g
Dietary Fiber: 0.8 g
Sugars: 0.4 g
Starches: 0 g
Protein: 0.4 g
Diabetic Exchanges: Free

Canola cooking spray
½ teaspoon canola oil
1 large yellow onion, coarsely chopped
2 stalks celery, including leaves, coarsely chopped
2 large carrots, coarsely chopped
6 cloves garlic, chopped
4 whole scallions, coarsely chopped
6 sprigs fresh parsley
2 sprigs fresh thyme
2 bay leaves
10 whole black peppercorns
1 small turnip, peeled and sliced
10 cups water

Heat a large stockpot over medium heat. Spray with cooking spray and add the oil. Add the onion, celery, and carrots and cook until the onion softens, stirring often, about 5 minutes.

Add the garlic, scallions, parsley, and thyme and heat for 1 minute, stirring. Add the bay leaves, peppercorns, turnip, and water. Bring to a boil over high heat. Reduce heat to low and simmer for 1½ hours.

Strain the broth into a second stockpot. Discard the solids. Use immediately, cover and refrigerate until ready to use, or freeze in various size containers for later use (we suggest sizes ranging from 1 to 4 cups).

French Onion Soup

French onion soup is definitely a classic, yet most people only eat it when they dine out. Unfortunately, restaurants usually load it with butter and salt. Our version is rich and savory and manages to keep the fat and sodium under control. The Gravy Master adds richness and can be found in most major supermarkets, but its omission will still result in a delicious soup.

1 teaspoon olive oil
1 teaspoon light margarine
6 yellow or Vidalia onions, sliced
2 tablespoons all-purpose flour
6½ cups Homemade Beef Broth (page 67), or
    reduced-sodium, low-fat beef broth
½ teaspoon Gravy Master
2 tablespoons dry sherry
6 thin slices of Italian bread, about ⅓-inch thick
6 slices reduced-sodium, reduced-fat Swiss cheese
2 teaspoons fresh parsley, chopped

In a large saucepan, heat the oil and margarine over medium heat. Add the onion and reduce heat to medium-low. Cook for about 20 minutes, stirring often, or until onions are soft and have caramelized.

Stir in the flour, then add the beef broth and Gravy Master. Cover and cook over low heat for 15 minutes. Add the sherry and continue to cook for 5 minutes. Divide the onions and broth among 6 broiler-safe soup bowls, making sure to leave about 1 inch of space at the top of each bowl. Top each with 1 slice of Italian bread and 1 slice of cheese. Broil until the cheese melts and starts to bubble. Remove from broiler, top with chopped fresh parsley, and serve.

YIELD: 6 servings, about 1 cup per serving

Nutritional Information Per Serving (1 cup):

Calories: 177
Fat: 4.6 g
  Saturated Fat: 2.1 g
  Monounsaturated Fat: 1.7 g
  Polyunsaturated Fat: 0.4 g
Cholesterol: 15 mg
Sodium: 102 mg
Carbohydrate: 20.1 g
Dietary Fiber: 3 g
Sugars: 0.2 g
Starches: 5 g
Protein: 12.9 g
Diabetic Exchanges:
  1 Starch/Bread, 1 Lean Meat,
  1 Vegetable

Gazpacho for Four

Perfect for a hot summer day, this refreshing, zesty tomato-based soup is served chilled and can be made a day in advance. For a Fourth of July theme, serve with a dollop of fat-free sour cream and a few blue tortilla chips in the center of the bowl of soup.

YIELD: 4 servings, about 1 cup per serving

¼ cup finely chopped red onion
2 cloves garlic, minced
¼ cup diced green bell pepper
1 medium cucumber, peeled, seeded, and diced
6 medium tomatoes, peeled, seeded, and diced
¾ cup Homemade Chicken Broth (page 66), or
    reduced-sodium, low-fat chicken broth
16 ounces tomato juice, no salt added
2 tablespoons red wine vinegar
2 teaspoons balsamic vinegar
2 teaspoons no-salt Italian seasoning
½ teaspoon salt substitute
¼ teaspoon freshly ground black pepper
1 teaspoon hot pepper sauce
2 teaspoons light sour cream
1 scallion, thinly sliced

**Nutritional Information
Per Serving (1 cup):**

Calories: 93
Fat: 0.9 g
  Saturated Fat: 0.1 g
  Monounsaturated Fat: 0.1 g
  Polyunsaturated Fat: 0.4 g
Cholesterol: 0 mg
Sodium: 258 mg
Carbohydrate: 20.1 g
Dietary Fiber: 3.8 g
Sugars: 6.3 g
Starches: 0.8 g
Protein: 4.8 g
Diabetic Exchanges:
  4 Vegetable

In a large bowl, combine all the ingredients except the sour cream and scallion, and stir well. Cover the bowl with plastic wrap and refrigerate until well chilled. Divide among 4 bowls and top each with ½ teaspoon sour cream and a sprinkling of scallion. This can be made a day in advance and kept in the refrigerator until ready to serve.

Hearty Chicken Vegetable Soup

This flavorful soup is chock full of vegetables and chicken and doesn't need a lot of salt or fat to taste good. Add some cooked rice or pasta to make it even heartier.

YIELD: 6 servings, 1 cup per serving

2 cups Homemade Chicken Broth (page 66), or reduced-sodium, low-fat chicken broth
4 cups water
1 pound skinless boneless chicken breasts, cut into bite-size pieces
3 tablespoons finely chopped fresh parsley, divided
Canola cooking spray
1 teaspoon olive oil
1 cup chopped onion
1 cup sliced mushrooms
1 garlic clove, minced
3 medium carrots, sliced
1 cup sliced celery
1 tablespoon cream sherry, optional
¼ teaspoon salt substitute
¼ teaspoon freshly ground black pepper
2 tablespoons frozen green peas, thawed

Nutritional Information Per Serving (1 cup):

Calories: 129
Fat: 2.2 g
 Saturated Fat: 0.4 g
 Monounsaturated Fat: 0.9 g
 Polyunsaturated Fat: 0.5 g
Cholesterol: 43 mg
Sodium: 93 mg
Carbohydrate: 8.2 g
Dietary Fiber: 2.4 g
Sugars: 0.5 g
Starches: 0.3 g
Protein: 19 g
Diabetic Exchanges:
 1 Medium-Fat Meat,
 2 Vegetable

In a 3-quart saucepan, bring the chicken broth and water to a boil over high heat. Add the chicken and 2 tablespoons of the parsley. Reduce heat to medium and simmer, uncovered, for 7 minutes.

Meanwhile, heat a large nonstick skillet over medium heat. Away from the heat source, spray with cooking spray and add the oil. Return to the heat, add the onion, and cook until softened, about 5 minutes, stirring occasionally. Add the mushrooms, garlic, and the remaining parsley and cook until mushrooms are tender.

Add the carrots, celery, mushroom mixture, sherry, salt substitute, and pepper to the simmering chicken and cook until the carrots are fork tender. Stir in the peas and cook for 1 minute. Serve hot.

Sausage Cannellini Soup

Cannellini beans are white beans widely used in Italian cuisine. You may find them sold as white kidney beans, and you can usually substitute Great Northern beans for them in recipes. Cannellini beans are an excellent low-fat source of protein, iron, and folate, and they provide about 6 grams of fiber per serving. This recipe calls for canned beans, but you can easily substitute dry beans that have been prepared according to the package directions.

YIELD: 6 servings, about 1 cup per serving

Nutritional Information Per Serving (1 cup):
Calories: 159
Fat: 5.8 g
  Saturated Fat: 1.8 g
  Monounsaturated Fat: 2.6 g
  Polyunsaturated Fat: 0.9 g
Cholesterol: 15 mg
Sodium: 375 mg
Carbohydrate: 18.2 g
Dietary Fiber: 4.8 g
Sugars: 0.9 g
Starches: 8.5 g
Protein: 8.4 g
Diabetic Exchanges:
  1 Starch/Bread, 1 Medium-Fat Meat

⅓ pound sweet or hot Italian sausage
Canola cooking spray
½ teaspoon olive oil
1 small onion, diced
1 clove garlic, minced
1 tablespoon tomato paste
2½ cups Homemade Chicken Broth (page 66), or
    reduced-sodium, low-fat chicken broth
3 cups water
1 14.5-ounce can low-sodium whole peeled
    tomatoes, chopped
1 15.5-ounce can low-sodium cannellini beans
1 teaspoon dried parsley flakes
¼ teaspoon dried basil
⅛ teaspoon dried oregano
⅛ teaspoon crushed red pepper flakes

In a heavy skillet, cook the sausage over medium heat until cooked through; poke several holes in the sausage with a fork as it cooks so fat can escape. Remove to paper towels and squeeze out as much excess fat as possible. Slice the sausage into ¼-inch slices, then cut each slice in half.

Meanwhile, heat a 2-quart saucepan over medium heat. Away from the heat source, spray with cooking spray and add the oil. Return to the heat, add the onion and sauté until soft, about 5 minutes. Add the garlic and cook for 45 seconds, stirring. Stir in the remaining ingredients and the sliced sausage, and heat until the soup simmers. Simmer for 10 minutes, stirring occasionally.

Hot and Sour Soup

This spicy soup is always a favorite at Chinese restaurants, and with good reason. It's spicy enough to get your attention and can serve admirably as an appetizer or as a meal. We think you'll be surprised when you find out how easy it is to prepare. It should take you less than 30 minutes to get it on the table. This recipe includes some ingredients that you may not be familiar with or have on hand, but they should be easy enough to find in most major supermarkets.

YIELD: 4 servings, about 1 cup per serving

**Nutritional Information
Per Serving (1 cup):**

Calories: 89
Fat: 1.9 g
  Saturated Fat: 0.4 g
  Monounsaturated Fat: 0.6 g
  Polyunsaturated Fat: 0.7 g
Cholesterol: 9 mg
Sodium: 554 mg
Carbohydrate: 11 g
Dietary Fiber: 1.1 g
Sugars: 0.6 g
Starches: 2.4 g
Protein: 7.8 g
Diabetic Exchanges:
  ½ Starch/Bread, 1 Very Lean
  Meat, 1 Vegetable

3 ounces pork loin
3½ cups Homemade Chicken Broth (page 66) or
  reduced-sodium, low-fat chicken broth
1 cup plus 2 tablespoons water
½ of an 8-ounce can sliced bamboo shoots
6 shitake mushrooms, sliced
1 clove garlic minced, about 1 teaspoon
1 teaspoon minced ginger
2 tablespoons reduced-sodium soy sauce
3 tablespoons rice vinegar
½ teaspoon ground chili paste
1 ounce Soba pasta (spaghetti-style), broken into
  2-inch-long pieces
2 tablespoons cornstarch
3 ounces firm tofu, drained, cut into ¼-inch
  cubes
Pinch ground black pepper
½ teaspoon sesame oil
2 scallions, sliced, green part only

Note: Most major supermarkets offer jars of peeled, sliced ginger in their Asian food aisle. We suggest using that for this dish. You should also be able to find ground chili paste in the same aisle. Both are inexpensive and work perfectly for this soup. Or you can substitute 1 teaspoon minced red chili pepper or ½ teaspoon crushed red pepper flakes for the ground chili paste. You can also use ½ cup dried, sliced shitake mushrooms instead of fresh, provided you soak them ahead of time according to the package instructions.

Trim visible fat from the pork loin; slice into ¼-inch wide strips.

In a large saucepan, heat the chicken broth and 1 cup water over high heat until it begins to boil.

Reduce heat to medium and add the pork, bamboo shoots, mushrooms, garlic, ginger, soy sauce, rice vinegar, and chili paste. Cover and simmer for 7 minutes. Add the Soba pasta and simmer for 3 minutes.

In a small bowl, stir the 2 tablespoons of water and cornstarch until smooth. Slowly stir the cornstarch mixture into the simmering soup. Continue to stir until the soup thickens slightly. Add the tofu and black pepper; simmer for 5 minutes. Remove from heat and stir in the sesame oil.

Ladle the soup into 4 bowls, top with sliced scallions, and serve hot.

Corn and Crabmeat Chowder

This recipe calls for frozen corn kernels, but you can use fresh corn if it is in season. You can steam, boil, or grill the fresh corn and shuck the kernels off. Grilled corn will lend a smokier flavor to the chowder. Imitation crabmeat also works well for this chowder, especially with the Mexican-Style variation.

Canola cooking spray
½ teaspoon olive oil
½ cup chopped yellow onion
1 small clove garlic, minced
1½ cups Homemade Chicken Broth (page 66), or reduced-sodium, low-fat chicken broth
2½ cups evaporated nonfat milk
1½ cups frozen corn kernels, thawed
¾ cup lump crabmeat or imitation crabmeat
¼ cup water
1½ tablespoons cornstarch
1 tablespoon chopped roasted red pepper
Freshly ground black pepper, to taste
Chopped fresh parsley, optional garnish

Heat a 3-quart saucepan over medium heat. Spray with cooking spray and add the oil. Add the onion

YIELD: 6 servings, about 1 cup per serving

Nutritional Information Per Serving (1 cup):

Calories: 151
Fat: 1.3 g
 Saturated Fat: 0.2 g
 Monounsaturated Fat: 0.6 g
 Polyunsaturated Fat: 0.3 g
Cholesterol: 21 mg
Sodium: 193 mg
Carbohydrate: 23.3 g
Dietary Fiber: 1.6 g
Sugars: 0.3 g
Starches: 0 g
Protein: 13.1 g
Diabetic Exchanges:
 1 Vegetable, 1½ Fat-Free Milk

and sauté until soft, about 5 minutes. Add the garlic and sauté for 1 minute. Add the chicken broth, milk, and corn and heat until it simmers for 5 minutes. Add the crabmeat and simmer for 5 more minutes, stirring often.

In a small bowl, combine the water and cornstarch and stir until smooth. Stir into the simmering soup and continue cooking until the soup thickens. Add the chopped roasted pepper and season lightly with freshly ground black pepper.

Divide the soup among 6 cups and garnish with chopped fresh parsley, if desired.

Variation
You can easily turn this into Mexican-Style Corn and Crabmeat Chowder by adding ½ cup fat-free salsa (or more to taste) along with the roasted red pepper.

Cream of Broccoli Soup

This is one of the most popular soups served in restaurants all across America. Unfortunately, it usually contains enough fat and calories to ruin most diets. This version is creamy, chunky, simple to make, and healthy. From start to finish, you can get this on the table in under 20 minutes. To reheat leftovers, add 1 tablespoon skim milk per 1 cup leftover soup and heat over medium-low heat until hot.

3 tablespoons all-purpose flour
1⅔ cups Homemade Chicken Broth (page 66), or
    reduced-sodium, low-fat chicken broth, divided
2 tablespoons fat-free cream cheese
1 10-ounce package frozen chopped broccoli, thawed
1 cup evaporated nonfat milk
½ cup skim milk
1 ounce shredded reduced-fat, reduced-sodium,
    mild white Cheddar cheese
Dash ground black pepper, or to taste
Pinch salt substitute
1 tablespoon chopped fresh parsley, optional
    garnish

YIELD: 4 servings, about 1 cup per serving

Nutritional Information Per Serving (1 cup):
Calories: 134
Fat: 1.1 g
    Saturated Fat: 0.5 g
    Monounsaturated Fat: 0.3 g
    Polyunsaturated Fat: 0.2 g
Cholesterol: 6 mg
Sodium: 160 mg
Carbohydrate: 19.8 g
Dietary Fiber: 2.6 g
Sugars: 1.7 g
Starches: 0.4 g
Protein: 12 g
Diabetic Exchanges:
    2 Vegetable, 1 Fat-Free milk

In a small bowl, mix 3 tablespoons flour with 3 tablespoons chicken broth until it is a smooth paste.

In a large saucepan, bring the remaining chicken broth to a boil over medium-high heat. Whisk in the flour paste and simmer until the broth thickens, whisking constantly, about 1 minute. Reduce heat to medium.

Remove ¼ cup hot broth from the saucepan and place in a bowl with the cream cheese. Stir together until smooth and return mixture to the saucepan. Stir in the broccoli, evaporated milk, skim milk, and cheese. Season lightly with pepper and salt substitute. Heat until hot and thickened, stirring often, about 5 minutes.

Ladle into small bowls, sprinkle with fresh parsley if desired, and serve hot.

Sherried Cream of Carrot Soup

Unfortunately, some of our readers still believe that carrots are a no-no for diabetics because they are sweet and full of sugar. This couldn't be further from the truth! Carrots are a great source of potassium and vitamin A and only contain about 6 grams of carbohydrate per serving. This wonderfully sweet soup reheats well in a saucepan or in the microwave. Make sure you cook the carrots and sweet potato until they are very soft; otherwise your soup will not have the smooth texture that it should have.

2 cups Homemade Chicken Broth (page 66), or reduced-sodium, low-fat chicken broth
2 cups water
2 cups sliced carrots
½ cup peeled and cubed sweet potato or yam
2 tablespoons minced Vidalia or other sweet yellow onion
⅓ cup skim milk
⅔ cup evaporated nonfat milk
1 tablespoon cream sherry
Pinch salt substitute
Pinch ground white pepper
4 sprigs fresh parsley, as garnish

In a large stockpot or saucepan, bring the chicken broth and water to a boil over high heat. Add the

YIELD: 4 servings, about 1 cup per serving

Nutritional Information Per Serving (1 cup):

Calories: 108
Fat: 0.3 g
  Saturated Fat: 0.1 g
  Monounsaturated Fat: 0 g
  Polyunsaturated Fat: 0.1 g
Cholesterol: 2 mg
Sodium: 364 mg
Carbohydrate: 18.4 g
Dietary Fiber: 2.7 g
Sugars: 0.9 g
Starches: 0.1 g
Protein: 6.5 g
Diabetic Exchanges:
  ½ Starch/Bread, 1 Vegetable, ½ Fat-Free Milk

carrots, sweet potato, and onion. Reduce heat and simmer until the carrots and sweet potato are very soft, about 10 minutes.

Carefully spoon the vegetables and broth, in small batches, into a food processor or blender and purée until smooth. Pour the puréed vegetables into a second large saucepan or stockpot and return to medium heat.

Once all of the vegetables are puréed, stir in the skim milk, evaporated milk, and sherry. Season lightly with salt substitute and ground white pepper. Continue to simmer for 7 minutes, stirring occasionally.

Ladle into bowls and serve hot with a parsley sprig floating in the center, as garnish.

Pasta e Fagiole Soup

This rich, savory, and absolutely delicious soup was inspired by a version served at Iannelli's Ristorante in Oneonta, New York. It will surely become a staple in your home during the cold-weather months. It freezes and reheats well and can be kept, covered and refrigerated, for up to 4 days.

YIELD: About 20 servings, about 1 cup per serving

1 4.5-ounce link reduced-fat Italian sausage, hot or mild
1 teaspoon olive oil
1 large yellow onion, chopped, preferably Vidalia
2 cloves garlic, chopped
2 6-ounce cans tomato paste
6 cups Homemade Chicken Broth (page 66) or reduced-sodium, low-fat chicken broth
4 14.5-ounce cans low-sodium Italian-style whole tomatoes
4 15.5-ounce cans cannellini beans, rinsed and drained
9 cups water
2 teaspoons dried parsley flakes
½ teaspoon no-salt Italian seasoning
Pinch ground black pepper
Chopped cooked pasta, 2 tablespoons per serving
Grated Romano cheese, 2 teaspoons per serving

Nutritional Information Per Serving (1 cup):
Calories: 159
Fat: 2.8 g
  Saturated Fat: 0.8 g
  Monounsaturated Fat: 0.6 g
  Polyunsaturated Fat: 0.5 g
Cholesterol: 7 mg
Sodium: 441 mg
Carbohydrate: 25.6 g
Dietary Fiber: 5.6 g
Sugars: 1.4 g
Starches: 14.9 g
Protein: 8.5 g
Diabetic Exchanges:
  1 Starch/Bread, 2 Vegetable,
  ½ Fat

Slowly cook the sausage over medium heat in a nonstick skillet until cooked through. Poke holes in the sausage while it cooks to let excess fat escape.

In a large stockpot, heat the olive oil over medium-low heat. Swirl the pot until the bottom is coated with the oil. Add the onion and sauté until soft, 7 to 10 minutes. Add the garlic and cook for another minute, stirring often.

Add the tomato paste and 1 cup of the chicken broth; stir until smooth (no tomato paste lumps left). Add the tomatoes and break them up with a wooden spoon. If the canned tomatoes contained whole basil leaves, remove them, mince them, and return to the soup. Stir in the remaining chicken broth, cannellini beans, water, parsley, Italian seasoning, and black pepper.

Pat the cooked sausage with paper towels and add to the soup. Raise the heat to medium-high and simmer soup for 1 hour. You do not want the soup to boil, so lower the heat a little bit if it does.

Prior to serving, remove the sausage from the soup and finely chop.

To serve the soup: Ladle 1 cup soup (with beans) into a soup bowl. Stir in 2 tablespoons chopped cooked pasta and ½ ounce chopped sausage. Top with 2 teaspoons grated Romano cheese and serve.

Brazilian Smoked Black Bean Soup

This soup was inspired by the national dish of Brazil, known as feijoada. Feijoada is a stew made with black beans, smoked sausages and meats, and regional spices served with rice. This soup uses smoke flavoring to mimic the flavor of smoked meat and is low in calories, fat, and cholesterol.

YIELD: 6 servings, about 1 cup per serving

Nutritional Information Per Serving (1 cup):

Calories: 173
Fat: 1.8 g
  Saturated Fat: 0.2 g
  Monounsaturated Fat: 0.6 g
  Polyunsaturated Fat: 0.7 g
Cholesterol: 2 mg
Sodium: 169 mg
Carbohydrate: 30 g
Dietary Fiber: 10 g
Sugars: 4.7 g
Starches: 13 g
Protein: 10.3 g
Diabetic Exchanges:
  1½ Starch/Bread,
  1½ Vegetable

1 teaspoon canola oil
½ cup diced yellow onion
2 tablespoons diced carrots
2 tablespoons minced garlic
5 cups Homemade Chicken Broth (page 66), or reduced-sodium, low-fat chicken broth
1 cup water
2 15.5-ounce cans low-sodium black beans, rinsed and drained
Pinch ground cayenne pepper
½ teaspoon ground cumin
1 tablespoon minced pickled jalapeño pepper
½ teaspoon dried oregano
½ teaspoon salt substitute
1 tablespoon orange juice
⅛ teaspoon liquid smoke
6 teaspoons fat-free sour cream
¼ cup thinly sliced scallions

In a 3-quart saucepan, heat the oil over medium heat. Add the onion and carrots and cook until the onion softens, about 5 minutes. Add the garlic and cook for 2 minutes, stirring often. Add the broth, water, beans, cayenne pepper, cumin, jalapeño pepper, oregano, salt substitute, and orange juice. Raise heat to medium-high and bring to a boil. Add the liquid smoke and reduce heat; simmer for 10 minutes.

Ladle two-thirds of the bean mixture from the soup into a food processor or blender and purée until smooth. Stir the purée back into the soup and return to medium heat for 3 minutes, stirring to blend.

Serve each bowl of soup topped with 1 teaspoon fat-free sour cream sprinkled with sliced scallions.

Tortellini Soup with Escarole

Some brands of tortellini, especially the "fresh" varieties offered in the refrigerated area of major supermarkets, are loaded with fat (including excessive saturated fats) and cholesterol. Make sure you read the food labels so you can choose the healthiest one. The sodium content for this recipe is low because we're using our homemade broth. If you choose to use canned broth, you can reduce the sodium content by replacing the 8 cups of broth with 5 cups of broth and 3 cups of water.

YIELD: 8 servings, about 1 cup per serving

Nutritional Information Per Serving (1 cup):
Calories: 121
Fat: 2.1 g
  Saturated Fat: 0.8 g
  Monounsaturated Fat: 0.4 g
  Polyunsaturated Fat: 0.2 g
Cholesterol: 14 mg
Sodium: 130 mg
Carbohydrate: 21.3 g
Dietary Fiber: 2.4 g
Sugars: 1.6 g
Starches: 0 g
Protein: 5.3 g
Diabetic Exchanges:
  1 Starch/Bread, 1 Vegetable,
  ½ Fat

Canola cooking spray
½ teaspoons olive oil
½ cup diced onion
2 cloves garlic, finely chopped
8 cups Homemade Chicken Broth (page 66), or reduced-sodium, low-fat chicken broth
1 9-ounce package frozen, reduced-fat cheese tortellini
2½ cups chopped escarole
1 teaspoon dry white wine
½ teaspoon no-salt Italian seasoning
Dash ground black pepper
3 tablespoons diced roasted red pepper
Grated Romano cheese, optional

Heat a 3-quart saucepan over medium heat. Spray with cooking spray and add the oil. Add the onion and sauté until softened, about 5 minutes. Add the garlic and sauté for 30 seconds. Add the broth and bring to a boil over medium-high heat. Add the frozen tortellini and cook for 5 minutes. Reduce heat to simmer and add the chopped escarole, wine, Italian seasoning, and pepper; cook for 6 minutes, then stir in the roasted red pepper. Ladle soup into bowls and sprinkle lightly with Romano cheese, if desired.

Carrot Salad

One serving of this simple salad contains just about enough beta-carotene for your body to convert into an entire day's worth of vitamin A, which plays an important role in vision, regulating the immune system, and promoting healthy bone and cell growth. Try adding ¼ cup diced red onion for a refreshing variation or add some golden raisins for sweetness instead.

1 tablespoon extra-virgin olive oil
1½ tablespoons lemon juice
Pinch salt
⅛ teaspoon freshly ground black pepper
2 cups shredded, peeled carrots

Whisk the oil, lemon juice, salt, and pepper in a large bowl. Add the carrots and toss. Serve immediately or refrigerate, covered, until ready to use.

YIELD: 4 servings, about ½ cup per serving

Nutritional Information Per Serving (¼ of recipe):

Calories: 76
Fat: 3.6 g
  Saturated Fat: 0.5 g
  Monounsaturated Fat: 2.5 g
  Polyunsaturated Fat: 0.4 g
Cholesterol: 0 mg
Sodium: 37 mg
Carbohydrate: 10.9 g
Dietary Fiber: 3.2 g
Sugars: 0 g
Starches: 0 g
Protein: 1.1 g
Diabetic Exchanges:
  2 Vegetable, 1 Fat

Corn and Black Bean Salad

Perfect for picnics and barbecues, this low-fat, no-cholesterol salad is easy to make and packed with flavor and healthful fiber. You can keep it in the refrigerator, covered, for up to 3 days.

1 10-ounce package frozen no-salt-added corn
  kernels, thawed and drained
1 15-ounce can black beans, rinsed and drained
¼ cup chopped green bell pepper
¼ cup chopped red bell pepper
2 tablespoons minced fresh parsley
2 scallions, sliced, green parts only
1 teaspoon canola oil
2 tablespoons lime juice
¼ teaspoon freshly ground black pepper

Toss all ingredients together in a large bowl. Cover and refrigerate for at least 2 hours before serving.

YIELD: 4 servings, about ½ cup per serving

Nutritional Information Per Serving (½ cup):

Calories: 179
Fat: 1.9 g
  Saturated Fat: 0.2 g
  Monounsaturated Fat: 0.6 g
  Polyunsaturated Fat: 0.9 g
Cholesterol: 0 mg
Sodium: 102 mg
Carbohydrate: 34.9 g
Dietary Fiber: 9.2 g
Sugars: 2.2 g
Starches: 10 g
Protein: 9 g
Diabetic Exchanges:
  2½ Starch/Bread

Greek Salad

While olives are high in fat, most of it is a monounsaturated fat called oleic acid that has been shown to help reduce blood cholesterol levels. By helping to prevent the oxidation of cholesterol, the nutrients in olives may actually help prevent heart disease.

YIELD: 6 servings

**Nutritional Information
Per Serving (⅙ of recipe):**
Calories: 113
Fat: 7.4 g
  Saturated Fat: 3.3 g
  Monounsaturated Fat: 3.1 g
  Polyunsaturated Fat: 0.6 g
Cholesterol: 17 mg
Sodium: 360 mg
Carbohydrate: 9.8 g
Dietary Fiber: 2.6 g
Sugars: 0.3 g
Starches: 0 g
Protein: 4.7 g
Diabetic Exchanges:
  2 Vegetable, 1½ Fat

1 tablespoon olive oil
3 tablespoons red wine vinegar
1 teaspoon dried oregano
⅛ teaspoon dried basil
Pinch dried thyme
¼ teaspoon freshly ground black pepper
5 cups iceberg lettuce, torn into bite-size pieces
5 cups romaine lettuce, torn into bite-size pieces
18 cherry tomatoes
1 medium cucumber, peeled, halved, seeded, and
   sliced
6 kalamata olives
4 ounces feta cheese, crumbled
1 green bell pepper, sliced into 6 rings

In a medium bowl, whisk together the olive oil, vinegar, oregano, basil, thyme, and black pepper.

In a large bowl, toss the lettuce, tomatoes, cucumber slices, bell pepper rings, and olives with enough dressing to coat well.

Divide the remaining ingredients, except the pepper rings and feta cheese, among 6 plates. Top each salad with crumbled feta cheese and a pepper ring.

Mediterranean Bean and Tuna Salad

Most diets encourage the reduction of fat consumption, but omega-3 fatty acids are one type of fat that has been shown to lower blood pressure and a type of fat in the blood called triglycerides. The American Heart Association recommends eating at least two servings per week of fish high in omega-3 fatty acids, such as albacore tuna.

3 small tomatoes, quartered
¼ cup chopped Vidalia onion or yellow onion
1 scallion, finely chopped
1 15.5-ounce can low-sodium cannellini beans,
    rinsed and drained
1 tablespoon chopped fresh Italian parsley
1 tablespoon olive oil
1 tablespoon lemon juice
1 teaspoon balsamic vinegar
1 teaspoon honey
1 garlic clove, minced
1 7-ounce can solid white albacore tuna, packed in
    water, drained and flaked

In a large bowl, combine the tomatoes, onion, scallion, beans, and parsley. In a small bowl, whisk together the olive oil, lemon juice, vinegar, honey, and garlic. Pour over the bean mixture. Add the tuna and toss.

YIELD: 4 servings

**Nutritional Information
Per Serving (¼ of recipe):**

Calories: 194
Fat: 4.3 g
  Saturated Fat: 0.5 g
  Monounsaturated Fat: 2.6 g
  Polyunsaturated Fat: 0.7 g
Cholesterol: 14 mg
Sodium: 387 mg
Carbohydrate: 20.7 g
Dietary Fiber: 5.1 g
Sugars: 2.7 g
Starches: 9.5 g
Protein: 17.4 g
Diabetic Exchanges:
  ½ Starch/Bread, ½ Very
  Lean Meat

Refreshing Spring Tabbouleh

Tabbouleh uses a grain called bulgur, which is cracked wheat that has been processed, precooked, and dried. This salad goes well with grilled chicken or shrimp, and is perfect for picnics and barbecues. Some people are afraid to use mint because they think their food will be overpowered by the taste, which couldn't be further from the truth. Don't be afraid of this recipe or of the fresh mint it calls for; you'll be glad you tried it.

YIELD: 6 servings

**Nutritional Information
Per Serving (⅙ of recipe):**

Calories: 112
Fat: 1.2 g
  Saturated Fat: 0.1 g
  Monounsaturated Fat: 0.6 g
  Polyunsaturated Fat: 0.3 g
Cholesterol: 0 mg
Sodium: 14 mg
Carbohydrate: 23.6 g
Dietary Fiber: 5.7 g
Sugars: 0.4 g
Starches: 15.7 g
Protein: 3.8 g
Diabetic Exchanges:
  2 Starch/Bread, 2 Vegetable

1 cup bulgur (cracked wheat)
2½ cups water
¼ cup minced red onion
⅛ to ¼ teaspoon ground allspice
10 fresh mint leaves, chopped (about 1½ tablespoons)
1 tablespoon chopped fresh parsley, or 1 teaspoon dried parsley flakes
¼ cup finely sliced scallions
1 small garlic clove, minced (about 1 teaspoon)
⅓ cup minced seedless cucumber
¼ cup minced carrots
2 tablespoons lemon juice
1 teaspoon olive oil
Pinch ground black pepper, or to taste
8 grape tomatoes, sliced in half lengthwise

Place the bulgur in a large bowl and stir in the water. Let stand for 60 to 90 minutes, or until the bulgur is softened and no longer crunchy, but al dente (taste a few grains to test).

Meanwhile, in another large bowl, stir together the onion, allspice, mint, parsley, scallions, garlic, cucumber, carrots, lemon juice, oil, and black pepper.

Drain the softened bulgur in a tight-meshed strainer or sieve to remove as much water as possible. Pat down with a towel or paper towels to remove excess moisture if needed.

Add the bulgur and tomato halves to the onion mixture and toss until well combined. Serve at once or chill and serve cold. Store in a sealed container, refrigerated, for up to 2 days.

Lemon-Garlic Salad

A very refreshing treat on a hot summer day, this salad is wonderful served for lunch or as an appetizer. It can be increased easily for any size gathering. Do not toss until ready to serve so the lettuce doesn't wilt and become overpowered by the lemon and garlic.

2½ cups red or green leaf lettuce
3 grape tomatoes
Dash ground black pepper
½ teaspoon minced garlic
1 tablespoon lemon juice
½ teaspoon olive oil
1 slice Italian bread or Garlic Crostini (page 61), optional

Toss all the ingredients in a large bowl until the lettuce is lightly coated. Serve with 1 slice warm Italian bread or Garlic Crostini, if desired.

YIELD: 1 serving

Nutritional Information Per Serving (1 salad):
Calories: 55
Fat: 2.7 g
  Saturated Fat: 0.4 g
  Monounsaturated Fat: 1.7 g
  Polyunsaturated Fat: 0.4 g
Cholesterol: 0 mg
Sodium: 19 mg
Carbohydrate: 7.2 g
Dietary Fiber: 3.1 g
Sugars: 0.8 g
Starches: 0.5 g
Protein: 2.9 g
Diabetic Exchanges:
  2 Vegetable

Soho Sirloin Salad

The flavor combination of blue cheese, red onion, and seared steak is really satisfying in this dish. Allowing the steak to sit for a few minutes after cooking helps keep it moist when you slice it. This recipe doubles easily.

6 ounces thick top round steak
Freshly ground black pepper
4 cups (tightly packed) green and/or red leaf lettuce
6 small cherry or grape tomatoes
⅓ cup thinly sliced red onion
¼ cup shredded carrots
2 tablespoons light blue cheese dressing

Place the steak on a large plate and season both sides liberally with freshly ground black pepper.

Heat a large nonstick skillet over medium-high heat until hot. Cook the steak for about 5 minutes per side until medium-rare, or longer if desired. Remove from heat and set aside for 5 minutes.

Meanwhile, toss the lettuce, tomatoes, onion, carrots, and blue cheese dressing in a large mixing

YIELD: 2 servings as an entrée

Nutritional Information Per Serving (1 salad):
Calories: 232
Fat: 8.5 g
  Saturated Fat: 2.9 g
  Monounsaturated Fat: 3.3 g
  Polyunsaturated Fat: 0.9 g
Cholesterol: 81 mg
Sodium: 245 mg
Carbohydrate: 8.4 g
Dietary Fiber: 3.2 g
Sugars: 0 g
Starches: 0 g
Protein: 30.1 g
Diabetic Exchanges: 4 Very
  Lean Meat, 2 Vegetable,
  1 Fat

bowl until the leaves are lightly coated with dressing. Divide equally between 2 dinner plates.

Once the cooked steak has set for 5 minutes, slice it into ½-inch-thick slices. Arrange the slices on top of each salad and serve immediately.

Sicilian Salad

The anchovies in this salad add outstanding flavor and help turn it into the savory salad it was intended to be. Serve with Garlic Crostini (page 61) for lunch or dinner. This recipe can be halved or doubled.

3 tablespoons House Italian Dressing (page 216)
6 cups mixed lettuce greens
12 cherry or grape tomatoes
½ cup shredded carrots
¾ cup thinly sliced red onions
4 pepperoncini peppers, seeded and chopped
4 anchovies, chopped
4 pitted medium green olives

Prepare the dressing.

In a large mixing bowl, toss all the ingredients until the lettuce is lightly coated with dressing. Divide equally among 4 dinner plates and serve.

YIELD: 4 servings

Nutritional Information Per Serving (¼ of recipe):
Calories: 81
Fat: 2.8 g
  Saturated Fat: 0.5 g
  Monounsaturated Fat: 1.5 g
  Polyunsaturated Fat: 0.5 g
Cholesterol: 4 mg
Sodium: 259 mg
Carbohydrate: 12.1 g
Dietary Fiber: 3.8 g
Sugars: 2.1 g
Starches: 0.2 g
Protein: 4.4 g
Diabetic Exchanges:
  2 Vegetable, ½ Fat

House Salad

This is an outstanding before-dinner salad. If you find that you are still hungry after meals, double the lettuce called for in this salad. Eating more lettuce is much better than taking seconds of your main dish and can help you reach the satiety you may feel you are lacking from your meal. Prepare the ingredients for this salad ahead of time and store in resealable plastic bags or containers so you can toss them together easily.

1 cup leaf lettuce
2 tablespoons shredded carrots
2 cherry or grape tomatoes
1 thin slice red onion
1 pepperoncini, not packed in oil, optional
1 tablespoon House Italian Dressing (page 216) or
  low-calorie Italian dressing
Freshly ground black pepper, to taste

YIELD: 1 salad, easily doubled

Nutritional Information Per Serving (1 salad):
Calories: 47
Fat: 2.3 g
  Saturated Fat: 0.5 g
  Monounsaturated Fat: 1.4 g
  Polyunsaturated Fat: 0.3 g
Cholesterol: 1 mg
Sodium: 27 mg
Carbohydrate: 6.6 g
Dietary Fiber: 2.0 g
Sugars: 0.4 g
Starches: 0 g
Protein: 1.9 g
Diabetic Exchanges:
  1 Vegetable, ½ Fat

Mound the lettuce on a plate and top with the shredded carrots, tomatoes, sliced onion, and pepperoncini, if desired. Spoon the dressing over the salad and season with black pepper to taste.

Caprese Salad

You can easily increase this recipe to accommodate any number of servings. This easy, delicious salad, enjoyable anytime, also makes a great presentation as an appetizer for guests, served with Garlic Crostini (page 61). Freshly picked tomatoes during the peak of the season make this a genuine treat.

¼ cup sliced roasted red peppers, not packed in oil
4 ¼-inch-thick slices vine-ripened tomato
4 small fresh basil leaves
1 1-ounce ball of part-skim fresh mozzarella, cut into quarters
2 sun-dried tomatoes slices, packed fresh with no oil, halved
½ teaspoon extra-virgin olive oil
Pinch salt substitute, optional
Pinch freshly ground black pepper

YIELD: 1 salad

Nutritional Information Per Serving (1 salad):
Calories: 132
Fat: 7.4 g
  Saturated Fat: 3.4 g
  Monounsaturated Fat: 3 g
  Polyunsaturated Fat: 0.5 g
Cholesterol: 16 mg
Sodium: 391 mg
Carbohydrate: 9.4 g
Dietary Fiber: 2.2 g
Sugars: 2.7 g
Starches: 0.7 g
Protein: 9 g
Diabetic Exchanges:
  3½ vegetable, 1 Reduced-Fat Milk, 1 Fat

Mound the roasted red peppers in the center of a salad plate. Arrange the four vine-ripened tomato slices around the peppers. Top each slice with a basil leaf and a piece of cheese. Place one piece of sun-dried tomato between each of the tomato slices; drizzle everything but the peppers with olive oil and season lightly with salt substitute, if desired, and black pepper.

Busy Tuna Salad

Perfect alone, on a salad, or between two slices of whole grain bread, this tuna salad has a lot of interesting textures and flavors, which is why we call it "busy." It's a terrific low-fat source of protein and omega-3 fatty acids and can be made in a matter of minutes.

2 6-ounce cans tuna packed in spring water
1 small reduced-sodium dill pickle, finely chopped (about 3 tablespoons)
2 tablespoons finely chopped yellow onion
¼ cup shredded carrots
¼ cup finely chopped celery
2 to 3 tablespoons fat-free mayonnaise

Combine all the ingredients in a bowl and mix until well blended. Chill, covered, until ready to use.

YIELD: 4 servings

Nutritional Information Per Serving (¼ recipe):

Calories: 100
Fat: 1.3 g
  Saturated Fat: 0 g
  Monounsaturated Fat: 0 g
  Polyunsaturated Fat: 0 g
Cholesterol: 0 mg
Sodium: 63 mg
Carbohydrate: 2.6 g
Dietary Fiber: 0.5 g
Sugars: 0.8 g
Starches: 0.7 g
Protein: 19.1 g
Diabetic Exchanges: 2 Very Lean Meat, 1 Vegetable

Balsamic Chicken Salad

Grilled chicken that has been lightly marinated in balsamic vinegar tops a bed of mixed greens for a refreshing and easy-to-prepare dish. Serve for lunch or dinner with a slice of Garlic Crostini (page 61). This recipe can be halved or doubled easily.

2 3-ounce boneless, skinless chicken breast fillets, visible fat removed
3 tablespoons balsamic vinegar, divided
Canola cooking spray
3 cups tightly packed green and/or red leaf lettuce
4 small cherry or grape tomatoes
¼ cup shredded carrots
Pinch salt substitute
Ground black pepper, to taste

Place the chicken and 2 tablespoons balsamic vinegar in a resealable plastic bag and seal; shift the chicken around with your fingers so the vinegar gets distributed evenly; refrigerate for 20 minutes.

Heat a nonstick grill pan (or an outdoor grill) to medium-high heat. Away from the heat source,

YIELD: 2 servings as an entrée

Nutritional Information Per Serving (1 salad):

Calories: 181
Fat: 3.3 g
  Saturated Fat: 0.9 g
  Monounsaturated Fat: 1.2 g
  Polyunsaturated Fat: 0.7 g
Cholesterol: 72 mg
Sodium: 78 mg
Carbohydrate: 9.5 g
Dietary Fiber: 2.2 g
Sugars: 3 g
Starches: 2.2 g
Protein: 28.2 g
Diabetic Exchanges: 4 Very Lean Meat, 2 Vegetable

spray pan with cooking spray (or coat outdoor grill rack lightly with canola oil) and return to the heat. Remove the chicken from the marinade and grill until cooked through. Discard all of the remaining marinade.

Meanwhile, toss the lettuce, tomatoes, carrots, and remaining 1 tablespoon balsamic vinegar in a mixing bowl until the leaves are lightly coated. Season lightly with salt substitute and black pepper and divide equally among 2 dinner plates.

Slice the chicken breasts into ¼-inch-wide strips. Arrange the slices on top of each salad and serve immediately.

Big Cobb Salad

According to the Brown Derby Restaurant in Hollywood, Robert Cobb, the original owner, created the Cobb salad in 1936 when he whipped it together using ingredients he found in the restaurant's icebox. While our version doesn't include all of the ingredients Mr. Cobb used, it is a satisfying reduced-fat rendition that serves well as a main dish.

1 6-ounce boneless, skinless chicken breast fillet
Pinch ground black pepper
Pinch dried parsley flakes
Canola cooking spray
4 cups green or red leaf lettuce, broken into pieces
3 tablespoons fat-free ranch dressing
1 large vine-ripened tomato, seeded and diced (about ½ cup)
2 tablespoons sliced black olives
1 cold hard-cooked egg, cut sliced into quarters
1 strip turkey bacon, cooked crisp, chopped, or ¼ cup diced avocado
2 ounces shredded low-fat Monterey Jack cheese

Season the chicken with the black pepper and parsley flakes.

Heat a nonstick grill pan over medium heat. Away from the heat source, spray with cooking

YIELD: 2 servings as an entrée

Nutritional Information Per Serving (1 salad):

Calories: 267
Fat: 8.4 g
  Saturated Fat: 2.9 g
  Monounsaturated Fat: 3 g
  Polyunsaturated Fat: 1.2 g
Cholesterol: 164 mg
Sodium: 538 mg
Carbohydrate: 14.3 g
Dietary Fiber: 2.8 g
Sugars: 1.6 g
Starches: 6.3 g
Protein: 33.2 g
Diabetic Exchanges: 4 Very Lean Meat, 2 Vegetable, 2 Fat

spray and return to the heat. Grill the chicken until cooked through.

Meanwhile, toss the lettuce with the dressing in a bowl until the leaves are well coated. Divide the lettuce between 2 dinner plates. Top each plate with half of the tomatoes, olives, egg, and bacon (or avocado).

Slice the chicken breast into ¼-inch slices and divide between the 2 plates. Sprinkle with the shredded cheese and serve.

Asian Cabbage Salad

Low-fat and low-carbohydrate, this crisp salad makes a perfect side dish for Asian-inspired grilled seafood, pork, or chicken. It is also quite refreshing as a warm weather salad and serves well for a picnic or barbecue.

2 tablespoons rice wine vinegar
½ teaspoon ground ginger
1/4 teaspoon sugar
2½ cups napa cabbage, shredded
½ cup grated carrots
¼ cup diced scallions
¼ cup diced red bell pepper
2 tablespoons chopped cilantro leaves

In a large mixing bowl, combine the vinegar, ginger, and sugar. Add the cabbage, carrots, scallions, red bell pepper, and cilantro and toss well. Cover and refrigerate for at least an hour before serving.

YIELD: 4 servings, about ½ cup per serving

Nutritional Information Per Serving (½ cup):

Calories: 27
Fat: 0.3 g
  Saturated Fat: 0 g
  Monounsaturated Fat: 0 g
  Polyunsaturated Fat: 0.1 g
Cholesterol: 0 mg
Sodium: 45 mg
Carbohydrate: 6.0 g
Dietary Fiber: 1.9 g
Sugars: 0.3 g
Starches: 0 g
Protein: 1.5 g
Diabetic Exchanges:
  1 Vegetable

Creamy Coleslaw

This coleslaw is fabulous with our Rotisserie-Style Roast Chicken (page 111), as well as traditional barbecued chicken and pork dishes. Unlike some of the coleslaws sold in supermarkets, this version is low in calories, fat, and carbohydrate, and it gets added sweetness from granulated fructose.

YIELD: 12 servings,
¼ **cup per serving**

**Nutritional Information
Per Serving (¼ cup):**
Calories: 16
Fat: 0.1 g
  Saturated Fat: 0 g
  Monounsaturated Fat: 0 g
  Polyunsaturated Fat: 0 g
Cholesterol: 0 mg
Sodium: 63 mg
Carbohydrate: 3.4 g
Dietary Fiber: 0.5 g
Sugars: 0.9 g
Starches: 0.6 g
Protein: 0.7 g
Diabetic Exchanges:
  1 Vegetable

¼ cup skim milk
3 3-gram packages granulated fructose
¼ teaspoon salt substitute
⅛ teaspoon freshly ground black pepper
3 cups finely chopped cabbage
½ cup finely shredded carrots
2 tablespoons minced yellow onion
½ cup fat-free mayonnaise
¼ cup low-fat buttermilk
¼ teaspoon celery seed
2 to 3 drops hot pepper sauce

Combine the milk, fructose, salt substitute, and black pepper.

In a large bowl, toss the cabbage, carrots, and onion. Stir in the milk mixture and mix until well combined.

In a small bowl, combine the mayonnaise, buttermilk, celery seed, and hot sauce. Add to the cabbage mixture and mix well. Cover and refrigerate for 3 hours, stirring well every hour. Using a slotted spoon, transfer to another bowl, leaving behind the thin liquid in the bottom of the bowl. Serve chilled.

7

Entrées

Boneless Chicken Cacciatore

Chicken Stuffed with Rice and Smoked Cheese

Spicy Thai Chicken

Roast Cornish Game Hens in Sonoma Sauce

Spicy Southwestern-Style Grilled Chicken

Hearty White Chili

Chicken Marsala

Chicken Souvlaki Plate

Roast Chicken with Black Raspberry Sauce

Pecan-Crusted Chicken with Dijon Cream Sauce

Chicken Stuffed with Artichoke Hearts and Sun-Dried Tomatoes in Lemon-Basil Sauce

Tri-Colored Lemon Peppered Chicken

Chicken Francese

Grilled Chicken Tostadas

Chicken and Cashew Stir-Fry

Grilled Chicken Parmesan over Penne

Rotisserie-Style Roast Chicken

West Coast Turkey Pita

Fiery Curry Tilapia

Crisp Cornmeal-Coated Catfish

Cajun Pan-Grilled Catfish

Citrus-Grilled Salmon

Salmon with Spinach and Ricotta

Lemon-Poached Salmon

Shrimp Scampi over Pasta

Tequila Shrimp

Garlic Shrimp over Couscous

Shrimp Jambalaya

Scallops au Gratin

Linguine with Herbed Porcini Clam Sauce

Baked Sole Dijon

Halibut Topped with Vidalia Onion and Raspberry-Balsamic Sauce

Orange Roughy with Sun-Dried Tomato Tapenade

Steak au Poivre

Salisbury Steak with Mushroom Gravy

Rustic Pot Roast with Vegetables

Tex-Mex Casserole

Classic Italian Meatballs in
Pomodoro Sauce

Veal Piccata

Mediterranean Grilled Lamb
Chops

Greek Gyros with Tzatziki Sauce

Apricot Grilled Pork Tenderloin

Italian Roast Pork

Spinach Mushroom Lasagne

Macaroni and Cheese

Greek-Style Orzo with Spinach
and Tomatoes

Penne à la Vodka

Stuffed Cabbage Rolls

Cajun Club Sandwich

Grilled Veggie Sandwich

Rachael Sandwich

Cornmeal-Coated Chicken
Sandwich

Chicken Cordon Bleu Sandwich

Meatball Heroes

In preparing this cookbook, we knew that main dishes deserved a great deal of attention and thoughtful consideration. New readers often tell us that their meals have become boring because they end up preparing the same few dishes over and over again. With this in mind, we created over fifty recipes for main dishes, ranging from simple to complex, that will surely bring an end to anyone's culinary doldrums. With this many recipes, you can serve a different main dish every night for almost two months straight. How's that for variety! We also took into consideration the real need for dishes that serve only one person, as well as dishes that are designed for two to four servings but can easily be doubled or expanded to accommodate a family dinner or dinner party.

You may notice that many of the recipes in this cookbook are influenced by Mediterranean cuisine. It's no secret that we enjoy Mediterranean-style food, but we also learned through a recent survey that Mediterranean cuisine ranked first among our readers as the favorite style of cooking. The good news is that a Mediterranean diet is considered by many to be one of the healthiest. It generally includes a variety of fresh vegetables and fruits, legumes, nuts, grains, moderate amounts of fish and dairy, and only small amounts of red meats. And while Mediterranean cuisine isn't necessarily low in fat, it is lower in saturated fat than most American diets. It includes the use of olive oil, which contains monounsaturated fats that don't raise cholesterol levels as saturated fats do.

We mainly use olive oil or canola oil, which is also low in saturated fat, and we reduce the amount of fat whenever possible by choosing leaner cuts of meat. Look at our Boneless Chicken Cacciatore, for example. It is a filling, full-flavored version of a classic Italian dish, but it has less than 4 grams of fat (only 0.6 grams are saturated fat). Our lineup of Mediterranean main dishes includes such favorites as Chicken Francese, Chicken Marsala, Veal Piccata, and Classic Italian Meatballs in Pomodoro Sauce, as well as more creative dishes such as Salmon with Spinach and Ricotta, Greek-Style Orzo with Spinach and Tomatoes, Penne à la Vodka, Linguine with Herbed Porcini Clam Sauce, and Chicken Souvlaki Plate.

Let's not get carried away, though. We have dozens of great main dishes for you to enjoy that are not even remotely Mediterranean in style. Shrimp Jambalaya and Cajun Pan-Grilled Catfish are New Orleans–style dishes guaranteed to get your mouth watering. There are southwestern-style dishes like Tequila Shrimp, Grilled Chicken Tostadas, and Spicy Southwestern-Style Grilled Chicken. There are French dishes like Steak au Poivre, Baked Sole Dijon, and Orange Roughy with Sun-Dried Tomato Tapenade. And, of course, there are favorites like Rustic Pot Roast with Vegetables and Rotisserie-Style Roast Chicken.

In addition to providing a collection of tasty main dishes that can bring excitement to the table, we paid close attention to nutritional content to make it easier to design an entire meal around them. Just pick out something that can fit into your meal plan, along with a side dish or a tossed salad, and get yourself cooking.

Boneless Chicken Cacciatore

Traditionally prepared using bone-in chicken, our version makes a full-flavored and filling dish using boneless chicken breast. Serve with a side of brown or white rice for a complete meal.

2 4-ounce boneless, skinless chicken breast halves, fat-trimmed
Canola cooking spray
½ teaspoon olive oil
¾ cup chopped yellow onion
1 clove garlic, minced
2 14.4-ounce cans low-sodium peeled whole tomatoes
¼ cup water
1 teaspoon dry red wine
½ teaspoon no-salt Italian seasoning
½ teaspoon dried parsley flakes
Pinch crushed red pepper flakes, or to taste
Pinch ground black pepper, or to taste
½ cup roasted red pepper, chopped

Cut chicken breast halves into 4 similar-size pieces.

Heat a large nonstick skillet over medium heat. Away from the heat source, spray with cooking spray and add the oil. Return to the heat, add the onion, and sauté until tender and golden, about 8 minutes. Add the chicken and sauté for 4 minutes. Add the garlic and sauté for 30 seconds.

Add the tomatoes, along with the juice, and the water. Stir in the red wine, Italian seasoning, parsley, crushed red pepper, and black pepper. Reduce heat to medium-low and simmer for 20 minutes, uncovered. Stir in the roasted red pepper and simmer for 2 minutes. Divide between 2 plates and serve hot.

Yield: 2 servings, can be doubled

Nutritional Information Per Serving (½ of recipe):

Calories: 252
Fat: 3.6 g
 Saturated Fat: 0.6 g
 Monounsaturated Fat: 1.3 g
 Polyunsaturated Fat: 0.8 g
Cholesterol: 64 mg
Sodium: 285 mg
Carbohydrate: 26.4 g
Dietary Fiber: 6.1 g
Sugars: 3 g
Starches: 0 g
Protein: 31.4 g
Diabetic Exchanges: 3 Very Lean Meat, 5 Vegetable, ½ Fat

Chicken Stuffed with Rice and Smoked Cheese

Moist chicken breast surrounds a blend of brown rice, sun-dried tomato, and smoked cheese for a dish that looks and tastes wonderful. You can use wild rice instead of brown rice and golden raisins instead of sun-dried tomatoes for a dish well suited for an autumn dinner.

Yield: 4 servings

**Nutritional Information
Per Serving (¼ of recipe):**
Calories: 255
Fat: 4 g
  Saturated Fat: 1.3 g
  Monounsaturated Fat: 1.2 g
  Polyunsaturated Fat: 0.7 g
Cholesterol: 68 mg
Sodium: 261 mg
Carbohydrate: 22.3 g
Dietary Fiber: 1.5 g
Sugars: 0.4 g
Starches: 10.1 g
Protein: 31 g
Diabetic Exchanges:
  1½ Starch/Bread, 4 Very
  Lean Meat

1 cup cooked brown rice
2 tablespoons chopped sun-dried tomatoes, fresh packed
1 tablespoon chopped fresh basil
¼ cup finely shredded smoked part-skim mozzarella cheese
⅛ teaspoon ground black pepper
½ cup unseasoned bread crumbs
2 teaspoons dried parsley flakes
4 4-ounce skinless, boneless chicken breast halves, fat trimmed, pounded to ¼-inch thickness
Canola cooking spray

Preheat oven to 350 degrees F.

In a large bowl, combine the rice, tomatoes, basil, cheese, and black pepper. Mix the bread crumbs and the parsley together in another bowl.

Lay the pieces of chicken out so they are flat and spoon ¼ of the rice mixture onto the middle of each piece. Roll each chicken breast, tucking in the sides, and secure with wooden toothpicks. Roll each stuffed chicken breast in the bread crumb mixture until lightly coated on all sides.

Line a baking pan with aluminum foil and spray with cooking spray. Lightly spray all sides of the stuffed chicken breasts with cooking spray and arrange them in the baking pan so they are not touching. Bake 25 to 30 minutes, or until chicken is cooked through, and serve.

Spicy Thai Chicken

Thai cooking includes ingredients such as lemon grass, ginger, garlic, coconut milk, curry, cumin, chili peppers, and basil. Fresh basil is a must for this Thai-inspired recipe, so don't even try to use dried basil. You can adjust the red pepper according to your taste. Serve with jasmine or basmati rice.

Yield: 4 servings

**Nutritional Information
Per Serving (¼ of recipe):**

Calories: 144
Fat: 2.8 g
  Saturated Fat: 0.5 g
  Monounsaturated Fat: 0.5 g
  Polyunsaturated Fat: 1 g
Cholesterol: 64 mg
Sodium: 209 mg
Carbohydrate: 2.4 g
Dietary Fiber: 0.4 g
Sugars: 0.7 g
Starches: 0.3 g
Protein: 26.5 g
Diabetic Exchanges: 4 Very
  Lean Meat

Canola cooking spray
1 teaspoon canola oil
4 4-ounce boneless, skinless chicken breast halves,
  fat trimmed
2 cloves garlic, minced
1 teaspoon ground chili paste, or ½ teaspoon
  crushed red pepper flakes
1 cup lightly packed fresh basil leaves, stems
  removed, thinly sliced
2 tablespoons lemon juice
½ cup cold water
1 tablespoon reduced-sodium soy sauce
½ teaspoon sugar
½ teaspoon ground black pepper

Heat a large nonstick skillet or wok over medium heat. Away from the heat source, spray with cooking spray and add the oil. Return to the heat, add the chicken, and brown on both sides. Add the minced garlic and chili paste and sauté for 1 minute.

Add half the basil along with the lemon juice, water, soy sauce, sugar, and black pepper. Stir well and cover. Reduce heat to medium-low and simmer, stirring occasionally, until the chicken is cooked through, about 5 minutes. Stir in the remaining basil, then remove the chicken to a platter and serve hot with the remaining sauce on top.

Roast Cornish Game Hens in Sonoma Sauce

Hens are roasted and served with a rich wine sauce complemented with smoked, sun-dried tomatoes. Serve with roasted or grilled vegetables and wild rice, if desired.

4 Cornish game hens, split in half down the back
Freshly ground black pepper
Canola cooking spray
1 cup diced carrots
¾ cup pearl onions, peeled
3 cloves garlic, sliced
2 teaspoons dried thyme
Pinch dried rosemary
2¼ cups Homemade Chicken Broth (page 66) or
  reduced-sodium, low-fat chicken broth, divided
1 cup California Zinfandel (or other full-bodied red
  wine such as Shiraz or Syrah)
1 cup low-sodium whole peeled tomatoes
3 tablespoons chopped fire-roasted sun-dried tomatoes, fresh packed

Yield: 4 servings

**Nutritional Information
Per Serving (¼ of recipe):**

Calories: 441
Fat: 10.3 g
  Saturated Fat: 2.6 g
  Monounsaturated Fat: 3.2 g
  Polyunsaturated Fat: 2.5 g
Cholesterol: 265 mg
Sodium: 261 mg
Carbohydrate: 15.2 g
Dietary Fiber: 3.3 g
Sugars: 0.8 g
Starches: 0 g
Protein: 60.7 g
Diabetic Exchanges:
  4 Medium-Fat Meat,
  5 Vegetable

Preheat oven to 425 degrees F.

Lightly season the hens with the black pepper. Place them in a large casserole or roasting pan. Spray the hens with cooking spray and roast until golden, about 20 minutes. Remove the hens from oven and lower oven temperature to 350 degrees F.

Heat a medium nonstick skillet over medium-high heat. Away from the heat source, spray with cooking spray. Return to the heat, add the carrots, onions, garlic, thyme, and rosemary, and sauté for 1 minute. Add ½ cup chicken broth and simmer for 5 minutes. Add the wine, the remaining chicken broth, and the whole peeled tomatoes and simmer for 10 minutes, stirring occasionally.

Spoon the sauce over the hens and return to the oven for 30 minutes, or until the hens are cooked through. Transfer the cooked hens to a large serving platter or to individual dinner plates, breast side facing up. Spoon any remaining sauce over each hen and sprinkle with sun-dried tomatoes. Serve immediately.

Spicy Southwestern-Style Grilled Chicken

Most of the ingredients from the marinade are also used for the seasoned black beans in this recipe. Make sure you read both ingredient lists so you can prepare everything at the same time. You can increase or decrease the level of heat by adjusting the amount of minced jalapeño pepper.

Jalapeño-Lime Marinade (page 214)
4 3-ounce boneless, skinless chicken breast halves, fat trimmed
Canola cooking spray
1 teaspoon olive oil
¼ cup chopped yellow onion
1 clove garlic, minced
1 15.5-ounce can low-sodium black beans, rinsed and drained
1 tablespoon lime juice
Pinch ground black pepper
1 tablespoon seeded, minced jalapeño pepper
1 tomato, seeded and chopped (about ½ cup)
2 tablespoons frozen corn kernels
1 teaspoon chopped cilantro
4 cups sliced or chopped iceberg or romaine lettuce
4 teaspoons light sour cream
1 scallion, sliced

Yield: 4 servings

Nutritional Information Per Serving (¼ of recipe):
Calories: 234
Fat: 3.6 g
  Saturated Fat: 0.7 g
  Monounsaturated Fat: 1.5 g
  Polyunsaturated Fat: 0.7 g
Cholesterol: 49 mg
Sodium: 161 mg
Carbohydrate: 23.5 g
Dietary Fiber: 8.3 g
Sugars: 1.9 g
Starches: 9.6 g
Protein: 27.8 g
Diabetic Exchanges:
  1 Starch/Bread, 3 Very Lean Meat, 2 Vegetable

Prepare the Jalapeño-Lime Marinade.

Place the chicken breast halves in a resealable plastic bag and add the marinade. Seal the plastic bag and shift the chicken around until it is well coated. Set the bag of chicken in the refrigerator for 1 hour.

Heat a 1-quart saucepan over medium heat. Away from the heat source, spray with cooking spray and add the oil. Return to the heat, add the onion, and sauté until tender, about 5 minutes. Add the garlic and sauté for 1 minute. Add the black beans, lime juice, and black pepper. Simmer for 2 minutes, stirring occasionally. Add the jalapeño pepper, tomato, corn kernels, and cilantro and simmer for 3 minutes, stirring occasionally. Set aside, covered.

Meanwhile, heat charcoal grill, gas grill, or grill pan to medium-high heat.

Remove the chicken from the marinade and grill until cooked through, discarding all of the remaining marinade. Serve the grilled chicken with bean mixture spooned over it and top with shredded lettuce, sour cream, and scallion.

Hearty White Chili

This is a great chili for football season because it only takes about 30 minutes to get on the table, plus it's a great way to use leftover chicken or turkey. You can also use this chili as a filling for burritos or tacos. Add more jalapeño or cayenne pepper for a spicier chili.

Yield: 8 servings, about ½ cup per serving

Nutritional Information Per Serving (¼ of recipe):

Calories:188
Fat: 3.1 g
  Saturated Fat: 0.4 g
  Monounsaturated Fat: 1 g
  Polyunsaturated Fat: 1.2 g
Cholesterol: 32 mg
Sodium: 183 mg
Carbohydrate: 19.7 g
Dietary Fiber: 5.7 g
Sugars: 1.6 g
Starches: 11.3 g
Protein: 19 g
Diabetic Exchanges:
  1 Starch/Bread, 2 Very Lean Meat, 1 Vegetable

1 tablespoon canola oil
1 medium onion, minced
1 clove garlic, minced
1½ cups Homemade Chicken Broth (page 66) or reduced-sodium, low-fat chicken broth
1 tablespoon chopped pickled jalapeño pepper
¾ teaspoon ground cumin
Pinch dried oregano
½ teaspoon cayenne pepper
⅛ teaspoon freshly ground black pepper
2 cups chopped cooked chicken or turkey
1 15.5-ounce can low-sodium white kidney beans
1 15.5-ounce can low-sodium red kidney beans

Heat the oil over medium heat in a large pot and sauté the onion until soft and golden, about 7 minutes. Stir in the garlic and sauté for 1 minute. Add the broth, jalapeño, cumin, oregano, cayenne pepper, black pepper, chopped chicken, and beans. Simmer for 20 minutes. If the chili seems dry, add additional chicken broth. Serve hot.

Chicken Marsala

This classic Italian dish gets its sweet flavor from Marsala, one of Sicily's most famous wines. This version is healthier than what is served in restaurants today, especially in terms of fat and sodium. Serve with rice or pasta, if desired.

¼ cup all-purpose flour
4 4-ounce boneless, skinless chicken breast halves, fat trimmed, pounded, ¼-inch thick
2 teaspoons olive oil
2 shallots, finely chopped
3 cups sliced white mushrooms
½ cup Homemade Chicken Broth (page 66) or reduced-sodium, low-fat chicken broth
¼ cup Marsala wine
1 tablespoon minced fresh parsley, or 1 teaspoon dried parsley flakes
Pinch freshly ground black pepper

Place the flour in a medium bowl and lightly dredge the chicken.

Heat the oil in a large nonstick skillet over medium heat. Add the chicken and brown, cooking for about 2 minutes on each side. Remove the chicken to a dish and set aside.

To the same skillet, add the shallots and sauté for 1 minute. Add the mushrooms and sauté until tender, about 5 minutes. Add the browned chicken (along with any juices that collected on the plate), broth, Marsala, parsley, and black pepper and simmer for 5 to 7 minutes, or until the chicken is cooked through. Serve hot, sprinkled with additional minced fresh parsley.

Yield: 4 servings

**Nutritional Information
Per Serving (¼ of recipe):**

Calories: 215
Fat: 4.2 g
  Saturated Fat: 0.8 g
  Monounsaturated Fat: 2.1 g
  Polyunsaturated Fat: 0.7 g
Cholesterol: 64 mg
Sodium: 80 mg
Carbohydrate: 11.1 g
Dietary Fiber: 1.1 g
Sugars: 0 g
Starches: 0 g
Protein: 29 g
Diabetic Exchanges: 4 Very Lean Meat, 2 Vegetable, ½ Fat

Chicken Souvlaki Plate

Souvlaki is a traditional Greek dish that features slices of roasted meat, such as lamb or beef, which are served in a pita with lettuce, tomato, onion, and Tzatziki Sauce. Our version turns something that is usually eaten like a sandwich into a filling salad for a lunch or dinner.

Yield: 4 servings

Nutritional Information Per Serving (¼ of recipe):
Calories: 213
Fat: 3.5 g
  Saturated Fat: 0.9 g
  Monounsaturated Fat: 1.4 g
  Polyunsaturated Fat: 0.7 g
Cholesterol: 66 mg
Sodium: 181 mg
Carbohydrate: 15.5 g
Dietary Fiber: 3.2 g
Sugars: 2.7 g
Starches: 0.3 g
Protein: 30.8 g
Diabetic Exchanges: 4 Very Lean Meat, 1½ Vegetable, ½ Starch/Bread

2 tablespoons olive oil
2 tablespoons lemon juice
1 teaspoon dried oregano
Pinch dried thyme
Pinch ground black pepper
1 pound boneless, skinless chicken breast, fat trimmed, cut into 1-inch cubes
4 tablespoons Tzatziki Sauce (page 210)
Canola or olive oil cooking spray
2 6-inch whole wheat pitas
8 cups iceberg lettuce, torn into pieces
16 grape tomatoes or 12 cherry tomatoes
4 black or green olives, optional
½ cup thinly sliced red onion

In a large bowl, combine 2 tablespoons olive oil, lemon juice, oregano, thyme, and black pepper. Add the chicken and set aside for 15 minutes, stirring occasionally.

Meanwhile, prepare the Tzatziki Sauce, if necessary.

Heat a grill or grill pan to medium heat.

Grill the chicken until cooked through, flipping occasionally. Set aside the chicken and raise the grill or grill pan heat to high. Spray both sides of the pitas with cooking spray and grill until golden on both sides. Cut each grilled pita into 6 wedges.

Divide the lettuce, tomatoes, olives, if desired, and onion among 4 large dinner plates. Top with the cooked chicken and serve with Tzatziki Sauce and grilled pita wedges.

Roast Chicken with Black Raspberry Sauce

This recipe is easy to make and it looks elegant when served. The rich plum-burgundy color of the sauce contrasts with the sliced chicken breast for a nice presentation. This is easy enough to make anytime, yet formal enough for any dinner party. If there are no fresh berries available, then you can leave them out.

Yield: 6 servings

**Nutritional Information
Per Serving (1/6 of recipe):**

Calories: 130
Fat: 2.4 g
  Saturated Fat: 0.7 g
  Monounsaturated Fat: 0.8 g
  Polyunsaturated Fat: 0.6 g
Cholesterol: 52 mg
Sodium: 51 mg
Carbohydrate: 6.5 g
Dietary Fiber: 1.6 g
Sugars: 2.8 g
Starches: 0.3 g
Protein: 19.5 g
Diabetic Exchanges:
  1 Medium-Fat Meat,
  1/2 Fruit

1 7-pound oven-roaster chicken
1¾ cups Homemade Chicken Broth (page 66) or
    reduced-sodium, low-fat chicken broth, divided
2 tablespoons all-purpose flour
¼ teaspoon Gravy Master
1 tablespoon black raspberry spreadable fruit
12 fresh blackberries
12 fresh red raspberries

Roast the chicken according to package directions. When the chicken is done, set it aside and prepare the sauce.

To prepare the sauce, heat 1½ cups chicken broth in a small saucepan over medium-high heat. Combine the remaining ¼ cup chicken broth with the flour in a small bowl and stir until smooth. Once the chicken broth begins to boil, whisk in the flour mixture and the Gravy Master. Continue whisking over medium-high heat until the sauce begins to thicken, about 2 minutes. Whisk in the black raspberry spreadable fruit and continue whisking until the sauce reaches the consistency of a light gravy. Set the sauce aside.

Remove the skin from the roasted chicken. Carefully remove each side of the chicken breast using a sharp knife to separate it from the bone. Place both pieces of chicken breast on a cutting board and slice each breast into ½-inch-thick slices.

Set out 6 dinner plates, preferably white. Pour 2 tablespoons of the black raspberry sauce into the middle of each plate. Swirl each plate until you have a thin round circle of sauce about 5 inches around.

Lay 3 or 4 slices of chicken breast (about 3.5 ounces per serving) in the center of the sauce on each plate. Drizzle each serving with 1 tablespoon of the sauce and garnish each plate with 2 blackberries and 2 raspberries.

Pecan-Crusted Chicken with Dijon Cream Sauce

Boneless chicken breast is coated with pecans and baked until crisp on the outside, while still moist on the inside. It is finished with a simple Dijon cream sauce and results in a savory dish with wonderful texture.

Yield: 4 servings

3 egg whites

2 tablespoons skim milk

4 4-ounce boneless, skinless chicken breast halves, fat trimmed

¼ cup ground pecans

2 tablespoons chopped pecans

Canola cooking spray

⅓ cup fat-free sour cream

2 tablespoons Dijon mustard

1 teaspoon dry white wine

¼ cup finely sliced fresh chives

Nutritional Information Per Serving (¼ of recipe):

Calories: 243
Fat: 10.1 g
  Saturated Fat: 1.1 g
  Monounsaturated Fat: 5 g
  Polyunsaturated Fat: 2.9 g
Cholesterol: 65 mg
Sodium: 320 mg
Carbohydrate: 6.3 g
Dietary Fiber: 1.2 g
Sugars: 3.0 g
Starches: 0.7 g
Protein: 31.3 g
Diabetic Exchanges: 4 Very Lean Meat, 1 Fat-Free Milk, 1 Fat

Preheat oven to 350 degrees F.

In a large bowl, beat the egg whites and milk. Add the chicken and stir until coated. Lay the coated chicken on a large plate in a single layer. Sprinkle both sides with the ground pecans, then press the chopped pecans into one side of each piece of chicken.

Place the chicken on a nonstick baking sheet with the chopped pecan side facing up. Spray with cooking spray and bake for 25 minutes, or until the chicken is cooked through.

Meanwhile, in a small bowl, mix together the sour cream, mustard, and wine. Set aside until ready to use.

Divide the cooked chicken among 4 plates with the chopped pecan side facing up. Top each serving of chicken with 2 tablespoons of sauce and sprinkle with chives. If you prefer a warm sauce, heat it briefly in the microwave before using.

Chicken Stuffed with Artichoke Hearts and Sun-Dried Tomatoes in Lemon-Basil Sauce

A lightly breaded boneless chicken breast is stuffed with artichokes, sweet sun-dried tomatoes, and fresh basil, topped with a light lemon-basil sauce, and served over angel hair pasta. You can use canned artichoke hearts, but they will most likely increase the sodium content.

2 4-ounce boneless, skinless chicken breast halves, fat trimmed

6 sun-dried tomato halves, fresh packed

3 ounces frozen artichoke hearts, thawed (about 1/3 of a 10-ounce package), cut into quarters, patted dry

2 fresh basil leaves

1/3 cup unseasoned bread crumbs

Canola cooking spray

4 ounces angel hair pasta or thin spaghetti

1 1/2 cups Homemade Chicken Broth (page 66) or reduced-sodium, low-fat chicken broth

2 tablespoons lemon juice

Pinch ground black pepper

3 tablespoons chopped fresh basil

Lemon slices

Yield: 2 servings

Nutritional Information Per Serving (1 stuffed chicken breast and 1/2 cup pasta with lemon-basil sauce):

Calories: 296
Fat: 3.1 g
  Saturated Fat: 0.6 g
  Monounsaturated Fat: 0.8 g
  Polyunsaturated Fat: 0.9 g
Cholesterol: 65 mg
Sodium: 292 mg
Carbohydrate: 34.3 g
Dietary Fiber: 4.4 g
Sugars: 2 g
Starches: 19.4 g
Protein: 32.9 g
Diabetic Exchanges:
  1 Starch/Bread, 1 Medium-Fat Meat, 5 Vegetable

Preheat oven to 375 degrees F.

Lay the chicken on a flat surface and flatten to 1/4-inch thickness. Place 3 sun-dried tomato pieces in the center of each piece of chicken. Top with pieces of artichoke heart and 1 basil leaf. Roll up each piece of chicken around the tomato-artichoke filling, tucking in the ends, and secure with toothpicks.

Place the bread crumbs in a bowl. Roll the stuffed chicken breasts in the bread crumbs until lightly coated on all sides. Spray the chicken on all sides with cooking spray and place in a baking dish that has been coated with cooking spray. Bake for 25 to 30 minutes, or until the chicken is cooked through.

Meanwhile, prepare the angel hair pasta al dente, according to package directions, without any added oil or salt.

In a medium skillet, heat the chicken broth over high heat until it begins to boil. Reduce heat to medium and add the lemon juice and black pepper. Simmer until reduced by one-third, stirring occasionally. Stir in the chopped basil and remove from heat.

Divide the pasta between 2 dinner plates and top each serving with 1 stuffed chicken breast. Divide the lemon-basil sauce between both servings, spooning it over the chicken and pasta. Garnish with lemon slices and serve immediately.

Tri-Colored Lemon Peppered Chicken

Three types of peppercorns are combined for a colorful and flavorful chicken dish well suited for spring and summer cookouts. There are commercial mixes available that already combine these three peppercorn types for use in a pepper mill that can make preparing this dish a little easier. This main dish goes along well with Lemon Couscous (page 175) and Grilled Vegetables (page 161) or Creamy Coleslaw (page 91) and Roasted Herbed Potatoes (page 169).

2 tablespoons canola oil
¼ cup fresh lemon juice
½ teaspoon coarsely ground or crushed red peppercorns
½ teaspoon coarsely ground or crushed black peppercorns
½ teaspoon coarsely ground or crushed green peppercorns
2 3.5-ounce boneless, skinless chicken breast fillets, fat trimmed
Lemon slices, optional garnish

Whisk the oil, lemon juice, and ground peppercorns in a medium bowl. Add the chicken and stir until coated. Cover and refrigerate for 1 hour.

Yield: 2 servings

Nutritional Information Per Serving (½ of recipe):

Calories: 126
Fat: 2.5 g
  Saturated Fat: 0.5 g
  Monounsaturated Fat: 0.8 g
  Polyunsaturated Fat: 0.9 g
Cholesterol: 56 mg
Sodium: 69 mg
Carbohydrate: 2.3 g
Dietary Fiber: 0.3 g
Sugars: 0.8 g
Starches: 1 g
Protein: 23 g
Diabetic Exchanges: 3 Very Lean Meat, ½ Fat

Heat an outdoor grill or nonstick grill pan to medium heat; lightly oil grill rack using a towel dipped in a little canola oil (or, away from the heat source, spray grill pan with cooking spray). Place the chicken on the grill and discard all remaining marinade. Grill the chicken until cooked through, 2 to 3 minutes per side. Serve garnished with lemon slices, if desired.

Chicken Francese

This is our light and flavorful version of the classic Italian restaurant dish, served over angel hair pasta with a fresh tasting lemon sauce. Not only do we love this dish, we love the fact that it isn't cooked in the oil or butter that usually loads it up with extra fat and calories.

Canola cooking spray
1 egg white
2 3.5-ounce skinless, boneless chicken breast halves, fat trimmed
2 teaspoons all-purpose flour
2 tablespoons unseasoned bread crumbs
1½ teaspoons dried parsley flakes, divided
4 ounces angel hair pasta or thin spaghetti
2 cups Homemade Chicken Broth (page 66) or reduced-sodium, low-fat chicken broth
¼ cup lemon juice
½ cup dry white wine
2 thin slices lemon

Yield: 2 servings, can be doubled

Nutritional Information Per Serving (½ of recipe):

Calories: 316
Fat: 2.8 g
  Saturated Fat: 0.6 g
  Monounsaturated Fat: 0.8 g
  Polyunsaturated Fat: 0.8 g
Cholesterol: 58 mg
Sodium: 182 mg
Carbohydrate: 31.9 g
Dietary Fiber: 2.2 g
Sugars: 2.0 g
Starches: 17.8 g
Protein: 30.1 g
Diabetic Exchanges:
  2 Starch/Bread, 2 Medium-Fat Meat

Preheat oven to 350 degrees F.

Line a baking sheet with aluminum foil and spray with cooking spray.

Place the egg white in a medium bowl. Add the chicken and move it around with a fork to coat it well.

Mix the flour, bread crumbs, and ½ teaspoon parsley flakes in a medium bowl. Lightly coat both sides of the chicken with the bread crumb mixture. Place the chicken on the prepared baking sheet and spray lightly with cooking spray. Bake for 20 minutes, or until the chicken is cooked through.

Meanwhile, prepare the angel hair pasta al dente, according to package directions, without any added oil or salt.

Heat the chicken broth in a medium skillet over high heat until it boils. Add the lemon juice and white wine and cook until the liquid is reduced by one half, stirring occasionally. Stir in the remaining parsley flakes and set aside until the chicken is done.

When the chicken is done, add to the warm lemon-wine sauce and stir to coat. Remove the chicken and serve each piece over ½ cup angel hair pasta drizzled with 2 tablespoons sauce. Garnish with lemon slices.

Grilled Chicken Tostadas

Grilled seasoned chicken and fresh vegetables rest atop a warm, crunchy baked corn tortilla in this classic Mexican dish. Finish it with sour cream, guacamole sauce, and a squeeze of lime and dive right in. Serve with a side of Refried Black Beans (page 166) or steamed rice, if desired.

2 3-ounce boneless, skinless chicken breast halves, fat trimmed
2 tablespoons fresh lime juice
Pinch ground black pepper
Canola cooking spray
2 6-inch corn tortillas
Pinch salt substitute
1 cup shredded lettuce
¼ cup diced, seeded tomatoes
2 tablespoons diced red onion
2 tablespoons nonfat sour cream
2 tablespoons Guacamole Sauce (page 210)
2 teaspoons thinly sliced scallions
2 teaspoons chopped fresh cilantro
Lime wedges

Preheat oven to 425 degrees F.

In a medium bowl, combine the chicken, lime juice, and pepper. Stir to coat; set aside.

Yield: 2 servings, can be doubled

Nutritional Information Per Serving (½ of recipe):

Calories: 201
Fat: 3.3 g
 Saturated Fat: 0.5 g
 Monounsaturated Fat: 1.3 g
 Polyunsaturated Fat: 0.8 g
Cholesterol: 49 mg
Sodium: 132 mg
Carbohydrate: 20.3 g
Dietary Fiber: 3.2 g
Sugars: 3.5 g
Starches: 10.9 g
Protein: 23 g
Diabetic Exchanges:
 ½ Starch/Bread, 2 Very Lean Meat, 3 Vegetable, ½ Fat

Spray both sides of the corn tortillas with cooking spray. Bake on a baking sheet until crisp and golden, but not brown, 5 to 7 minutes. Remove to paper towels and sprinkle both sides with salt substitute.

Meanwhile, heat a grill pan or grill over medium-high heat. Away from the heat source, spray lightly with cooking spray or lightly coat a grill rack with canola oil using a towel. Grill the chicken until cooked through, about 3 minutes per side, and discard all remaining marinade. Cut the chicken into ¼-inch-thick slices.

Place 1 crisp tortilla shell on each plate and top with shredded lettuce, tomatoes, onion, and grilled chicken. Top with sour cream and Guacamole Sauce and sprinkle with scallions and cilantro. Garnish with lime wedges.

Chicken and Cashew Stir-Fry

Our savory version of the Chinese restaurant favorite offers the same crunchy texture, while dramatically reducing overall fat and sodium content. You can use a large nonstick skillet if you don't have a wok, but your cooking times may not be the same. If you are in the mood for something spicy, add ½ teaspoon crushed red pepper flakes or ground chili paste when you add the soy sauce. Serve with steamed rice, if desired.

Canola cooking spray
1 teaspoon canola oil, divided
1 medium yellow onion, diced (about 1 cup)
1 cup diced carrots
⅔ cup diced celery
1 5-ounce can diced water chestnuts
2 cloves garlic, minced
6 ounces boneless, skinless chicken breast, fat trimmed, cut into small pieces
1 tablespoon reduced-sodium soy sauce
1 tablespoon water
3 tablespoons unsalted cashews, chopped
¼ teaspoon sesame oil

Yield: 2 servings

Nutritional Information Per Serving (½ of recipe):

Calories: 304
Fat: 11 g
  Saturated Fat: 2.2 g
  Monounsaturated Fat: 5.4 g
  Polyunsaturated Fat: 2.9 g
Cholesterol: 48 mg
Sodium: 656 mg
Carbohydrate: 28.6 g
Dietary Fiber: 6.2 g
Sugars: 9.9 g
Starches: 6.9 g
Protein: 25 g
Diabetic Exchanges: 5 Very Lean Meat, 2 Fat

Heat a wok over medium-high heat. Away from the heat source, spray with cooking spray and add ½ teaspoon oil. Return to the heat, add the onion, and stir-fry for 4 minutes. Add the carrots and celery and stir-fry for 3 minutes. Add the water chestnuts and garlic and stir-fry for 1 minute. Remove the vegetables to a bowl and set aside.

Add the remaining ½ teaspoon canola oil to the wok. Add the chicken and stir-fry for 4 minutes. Add the soy sauce and water and stir-fry for another minute. Add the cashews and toss with the chicken. Once the chicken is cooked through, toss with the sesame oil. Return the vegetables to the wok and toss with the chicken and cashews until thoroughly heated.

Grilled Chicken Parmesan over Penne

Usually Chicken Parmesan is fried in oil or sautéed in butter. We grill boneless chicken breast and serve it over penne with fresh basil and grated Parmesan cheese. The result is a much healthier dish that's actually easier to prepare and every bit as delicious.

Yield: 4 servings

Nutritional Information Per Serving (¼ of recipe):

Calories: 275
Fat: 3.5 g
  Saturated Fat: 1.1 g
  Monounsaturated Fat: 1 g
  Polyunsaturated Fat: 0.7 g
Cholesterol: 67 mg
Sodium: 195 mg
Carbohydrate: 27.9 g
Dietary Fiber: 3 g
Sugars: 2.4 g
Starches: 17.7 g
Protein: 32.4 g
Diabetic Exchanges:
  1½ Starch/Bread, 4 Very
  Lean Meat

8 ounces dry penne pasta
Canola cooking spray
4 4-ounce boneless, skinless chicken breast halves, fat trimmed, pounded to no more than ½ inch thick
2 cups Nona's Italian Marinara Sauce (page 205) or reduced-fat, reduced-sodium marinara sauce
3 tablespoons freshly grated Parmesan cheese
2 to 3 tablespoons chopped fresh basil leaves

Cook the penne according to package directions until al dente, without any added oil or salt.

Meanwhile, heat a nonstick grill pan (or grill) to medium-high heat. Away from the heat source, spray the pan with cooking spray and return to the heat. Grill the chicken until thoroughly cooked. Remove the chicken to a cutting board and cut into ¼-inch-wide strips.

Divide the cooked penne among 4 plates and top each with 4 ounces of sliced grilled chicken and ½ cup of marinara sauce. Sprinkle each with Parmesan cheese and fresh basil and serve immediately.

Rotisserie-Style Roast Chicken

Traditionally, rotisserie-style chicken spins while it cooks, basting itself with its own fat and juices as it rotates. Our version is seasoned without salt and is lower in fat because we remove the skin before cooking. The final step involving the broth makes the end result juicy and delicious. Served with a low-fat buttermilk biscuit and our Creamy Coleslaw (page 91), it's finger-licking good.

¾ teaspoon no-salt Italian seasoning
¼ teaspoon garlic powder
⅛ teaspoon onion powder
Pinch paprika
Pinch cayenne pepper
Pinch ground black pepper
⅛ teaspoon salt substitute
¼ teaspoon dried parsley flakes
8 split chicken breasts (about 3½ pounds), skin removed, fat trimmed
Canola cooking spray
1 cup Homemade Chicken Broth (page 66) or reduced-sodium, low-fat chicken broth

Yield: 8 servings

Nutritional Information Per Serving (one 7-ounce chicken breast):

Calories: 142
Fat: 1.9 g
 Saturated Fat: 0.5 g
 Monounsaturated Fat: 0.5 g
 Polyunsaturated Fat: 0.5 g
Cholesterol: 72 mg
Sodium: 84 mg
Carbohydrate: 0.5 g
Dietary Fiber: 0 g
Sugars: 0 g
Starches: 0 g
Protein: 29.4 g
Diabetic Exchanges: 4 Very
 Lean Meat

Preheat oven to 350 degrees F.

Combine the Italian seasoning, garlic powder, onion powder, paprika, cayenne, black pepper, salt substitute, and parsley flakes in a medium bowl. Rub this seasoning mixture into the meaty side of each chicken breast and arrange in a roasting pan with the seasoned side up. Spray the chicken with cooking spray and bake for 25 minutes, or until the chicken is cooked through.

Heat the chicken broth in a skillet over high heat until it begins to boil. Remove from the heat and dip the seasoned side of each cooked chicken breast into the hot broth for 10 seconds, then arrange on a large serving plate and serve.

West Coast Turkey Pita

Only use sun-dried tomatoes that are fresh packed, not those packed in oil. They are now readily available in supermarkets and often come packaged in a pouch or in the bulk food section. If they are hard, cover with hot water in a bowl and soak until softened but still firm.

½ cup Creamy Coleslaw (page 91) or low-fat, sugar-free creamy coleslaw
2 tablespoons chopped fresh-packed sun-dried tomatoes, softened if necessary
1 tablespoon golden raisins
1 8-inch whole wheat pita bread
Red or green leaf lettuce
3½ ounces low-sodium, low-fat, deli-sliced turkey breast or smoked turkey breast

Prepare the coleslaw, if necessary.

In a small bowl, mix the coleslaw, sun-dried tomatoes, and raisins; set aside.

Cut the top inch off of the pita and open carefully to expose the pocket inside. Place the lettuce in the pita pocket and top with the sliced turkey breast. Spoon the coleslaw mixture on top of the turkey and serve.

Yield: 1 serving, can be doubled

Nutritional Information Per Serving (1 pita):

Calories: 327
Fat: 2.5 g
  Saturated Fat: 0.3 g
  Monounsaturated Fat: 0.4 g
  Polyunsaturated Fat: 0.9 g
Cholesterol: 63 mg
Sodium: 780 mg
Carbohydrate: 45 g
Dietary Fiber: 4.1 g
Sugars: 2.9 g
Starches: 26.6 g
Protein: 30.4 g
Diabetic Exchanges:
  2 Starch/Bread, 3 Very Lean Meat, 1 Vegetable

Fiery Curry Tilapia

Tilapia is a firm, flaky type of fish with a sweet, mild flavor that can be found fresh or frozen in many supermarkets. The fillets are usually small, which makes portion control even easier. This can be served with white medium-grain rice along with steamed broccoli for a great low-fat meal.

Yield: 2 servings

**Nutritional Information
Per Serving (½ of recipe):**

Calories: 141
Fat: 2 g
  Saturated Fat: 0.5 g
  Monounsaturated Fat: 0.5 g
  Polyunsaturated Fat: 0.7 g
Cholesterol: 95 mg
Sodium: 559 mg
Carbohydrate: 1.7 g
Dietary Fiber: 0.3 g
Sugars: 0 g
Starches: 0 g
Protein: 27.3 g
Diabetic Exchanges: 4 Very
  Lean Meat

2 teaspoon fresh ginger, minced
¼ teaspoon curry powder
¼ teaspoon ground cayenne pepper
⅛ teaspoon crushed red pepper flakes
Dash ground black pepper
1½ tablespoons reduced-sodium soy sauce
2½ tablespoons water
Canola cooking spray
2 4-ounce tilapia fillets (or other similar white fish, such as cod or haddock)

Preheat oven to 400 degrees F.

In a small bowl, combine the ginger, curry, cayenne, red pepper flakes, black pepper, soy sauce, and water.

Line a baking dish with aluminum foil and spray with cooking spray. Place both tilapia fillets in the center of the foil and fold the foil right up to the edge of the fish until you have a 2-inch foil rim around the fish. Spoon the soy sauce mixture directly over each fillet. Bake for 7 to 9 minutes, or until the fish is cooked and crisp around the edges.

Crisp Cornmeal-Coated Catfish

Crisp on the outside and moist on the inside, this baked fish can be served with a little Cajun Tartar Sauce (page 208), Creamy Coleslaw (page 91), and a steamed vegetable for a wonderful meal. You can substitute similar types of fish, such as haddock, for the catfish, if you wish.

⅓ cup yellow cornmeal
2 tablespoons grated Parmesan cheese
2 teaspoons all-purpose flour
1 teaspoon dried parsley flakes
⅛ teaspoon freshly ground black pepper
⅛ teaspoon cayenne pepper
Canola cooking spray
4 4-ounce catfish fillets, about ½-inch thick

Preheat oven to 375 degrees F.

Combine the cornmeal, Parmesan cheese, flour, parsley flakes, black pepper, and cayenne in a mixing bowl.

Lightly spray a baking dish large enough to accommodate the four fish fillets with cooking spray.

Press the cornmeal mixture into the top of each fillet so that the each one is coated. Arrange the fish in a single layer in the baking dish, seasoned side up, and spray the top of each one lightly with cooking spray. Bake for 8 minutes, or until the fish is cooked through, and serve immediately.

Yield: 4 servings

**Nutritional Information
Per Serving (¼ of recipe):**

Calories: 201
Fat: 9.7 g
  Saturated Fat: 2.5 g
  Monounsaturated Fat: 4.4 g
  Polyunsaturated Fat: 1.9 g
Cholesterol: 55 mg
Sodium: 110 mg
Carbohydrate: 7.9 g
Dietary Fiber: 0.7 g
Sugars: 0 g
Starches: 0 g
Protein: 19.5 g
Diabetic Exchanges:
  ½ Starch/Bread, 2 Medium-
  Fat Meat

Cajun Pan-Grilled Catfish

For this dish, sometimes referred to as "blackened" cat-fish in restaurants, the fillets are coated with Cajun sea-soning and cooked until the seasonings blacken and crisp on the outside. Make sure you have your overhead fan turned on when cooking this dish, as it can create quite a bit of eye-watering smoke, courtesy of the spices.

4 4-ounce catfish fillets
Canola cooking spray
1 tablespoon No-Salt Cajun Spice Mix (page 215),
    or commercial reduced or no-sodium Cajun
    seasoning blend
1 medium lemon, cut into 8 wedges

Lay the fish out on a large plate. Spray both sides of the fish with cooking spray and press the No-Salt Cajun Spice Mix into each piece with the back of a spoon.

Heat a large skillet over high heat. Away from the heat source, spray with cooking spray. Return to the heat and add the fish. Cook for 3 to 4 minutes per side, or until the fish is firm and cooked through and the seasonings have black-ened slightly. Garnish with lemon wedges and serve.

Yield: 4 servings

**Nutritional Information
Per Serving (¼ of recipe):**

Calories: 153
Fat: 8.6 g
  Saturated Fat: 2 g
  Monounsaturated Fat: 4.1 g
  Polyunsaturated Fat: 1.8 g
Cholesterol: 53 mg
Sodium: 60 mg
Carbohydrate: 0 g
Dietary Fiber: 0 g
Sugars: 0 g
Starches: 0 g
Protein: 17.6 g
Diabetic Exchanges:
  2 Medium-Fat Meat

Citrus-Grilled Salmon

This recipe works well for outdoor grilling as well as broiling in the oven. The American Heart Association recommends that eating three servings of fish per week benefits our health, and may help reduce the risk of heart disease. If you are concerned about mercury content, then ocean-caught salmon is a better choice than farm-raised salmon. You can still reap the health benefits by choosing fish such as salmon, haddock, sole, cod, pollock, or tilapia instead of predatory fish such as shark, swordfish, and king mackerel.

¼ cup orange juice
⅔ cup lime juice
1 teaspoon olive oil
¼ teaspoon freshly ground black pepper
4 3-ounce salmon steaks, about ¾-inch thick
2 tablespoons sliced scallions
2 tablespoons water
1 teaspoon honey
Canola cooking spray

Yield: 4 servings

Nutritional Information Per Serving (¼ of recipe):
Calories: 190
Fat: 10.4 g
  Saturated Fat: 2 g
  Monounsaturated Fat: 4.1 g
  Polyunsaturated Fat: 3.5 g
Cholesterol: 50 mg
Sodium: 52 mg
Carbohydrate: 7 g
Dietary Fiber: 0.3 g
Sugars: 3 g
Starches: 0 g
Protein: 17.3 g
Diabetic Exchanges: 2 High-Fat Meat

In a small bowl, combine the orange juice, lime juice, olive oil, and pepper.

Place the salmon in a shallow dish. Pour all but 2 tablespoons of the juice mixture over the fish, and reserve the rest of the juice. Turn the fish to coat all sides and marinate for 20 minutes in the refrigerator, turning once after 10 minutes.

Add the scallions, water, and honey to the reserved 2 tablespoons juice mixture, and set aside. You will use this dressing to top the salmon after it is grilled.

To Grill: Heat grill to medium-high heat. Place each salmon fillet on the grill and top each with a few teaspoons of the marinade. Discard remaining marinade. Grill for 3 to 4 minutes per side, or until cooked through.

To Broil: Heat broiler with broiler pan in the oven positioned about 7 inches from the heat source. Remove preheated broiler pan and lightly spray with cooking spray. Place the salmon on the pan, skin side down, and top with a few teaspoons of the marinade. Discard remaining marinade. Broil for 7 to 10 minutes, or until fish is cooked through.

Drizzle each piece of salmon with 2 teaspoons of the citrus sauce you set aside earlier and serve hot.

Salmon with Spinach and Ricotta

Poached salmon is topped with a delicious combination of spinach, basil, and ricotta cheese for a filling meal packed with omega-3 fatty acids, protein, and folic acid. Poaching the salmon preserves moistness without added fat. You can use fresh spinach for this dish instead of frozen.

1 10-ounce package frozen chopped spinach, thawed
4 4-ounce salmon fillets
1 teaspoon olive oil
1 shallot, minced
3 tablespoons chopped fresh basil
¼ cup water
2 tablespoons dry white wine
½ cup part-skim ricotta cheese
2 tablespoons fat-free sour cream
Pinch salt substitute
Pinch ground black pepper
4 lemon wedges

Yield: 4 servings

Nutritional Information Per Serving (¼ of recipe):

Calories: 278
Fat: 13.3 g
  Saturated Fat: 1.7 g
  Monounsaturated Fat: 6.3 g
  Polyunsaturated Fat: 2.3 g
Cholesterol: 82 mg
Sodium: 148 mg
Carbohydrate: 7.5 g
Dietary Fiber: 1.9 g
Sugars: 1 g
Starches: 1.4 g
Protein: 29.8 g
Diabetic Exchanges:
  3 Medium-Fat Meat,
  2 Vegetable

Squeeze the thawed spinach until you have removed as much of the liquid as possible.

Fill a large nonstick skillet with 1 inch of water and bring to a boil over high heat. Add the salmon to the skillet in one layer, skin side down. Reduce heat to medium-low, cover, and poach until cooked through.

Meanwhile, in a medium nonstick skillet, heat the oil over medium heat. Add the shallot and sauté until softened, about 2 minutes. Add the basil, water, and white wine and simmer for 1 minute. Add the spinach, ricotta cheese, and sour cream and stir until well combined and heated through. Season with salt substitute and black pepper and set aside, covered.

Divide the poached salmon among 4 plates and sprinkle each with the juice of 1 lemon wedge. Top with the spinach mixture and serve.

Lemon-Poached Salmon

Moist salmon is delicately flavored with lemon for a light entrée that is simple to prepare. You can serve this with steamed string beans and a serving of brown rice for a well-rounded meal.

¾ cup white wine
1¼ cups water
2 tablespoons lemon juice
Pinch freshly ground black pepper
4 4-ounce salmon fillets
6 lemon slices
Fresh parsley sprigs

In a large skillet, heat the wine, water, lemon juice, and black pepper over medium-high heat until it begins to boil. Add the salmon fillets in one layer, skin side down, and add 2 lemon slices. Reduce heat to medium, cover, and poach for 5 to 7 minutes, or until the salmon flakes easily with a fork. Carefully remove the cooked salmon using a slotted spatula and serve immediately with a lemon slice and sprig of parsley on top of each fillet.

Yield: 4 servings

Nutritional Information Per Serving (¼ of recipe):

Calories: 235
Fat: 9.6 g
  Saturated Fat: 0 g
  Monounsaturated Fat: 4.8 g
  Polyunsaturated Fat: 2 g
Cholesterol: 72 mg
Sodium: 58 mg
Carbohydrate: 1.5 g
Dietary Fiber: 0.3 g
Sugars: 0 g
Starches: 0 g
Protein: 24.2 g
Diabetic Exchanges:
  3 Medium-Fat Meat

Shrimp Scampi over Pasta

The word scampi *actually means shrimp in Italian, making the name for the popular dish a bit ridiculous when you think about it. Nevertheless, ask most people what the* scampi *in shrimp scampi means and they'll probably say butter, garlic, or a combination of both. In this dish, shrimp are sautéed with garlic, lemon, and wine and finished with bread crumbs and fresh parsley before being served over linguine. Some people like to leave the tail on the shrimp instead of peeling it off, but we prefer to remove the entire shell, including the tail, to avoid any problems with errant pieces of shell.*

8 ounces dry linguine or angel hair pasta
1 tablespoon light margarine
1 teaspoon olive oil
1 pound medium shrimp, peeled and deveined
4 cloves garlic, peeled and finely chopped
1 tablespoon fresh lemon juice
⅓ cup dry white wine
¼ cup water
Pinch salt substitute
Pinch freshly ground black pepper
2 tablespoons chopped fresh parsley
1 tablespoon dry bread crumbs
4 lemon wedges, optional

Yield: 4 servings

**Nutritional Information
Per Serving (¼ of recipe):**

Calories: 233
Fat: 4.7 g
　Saturated Fat: 0.4 g
　Monounsaturated Fat: 1.8 g
　Polyunsaturated Fat: 1.4 g
Cholesterol: 134 mg
Sodium: 174 mg
Carbohydrate: 22.5 g
Dietary Fiber: 1.1 g
Sugars: 2.4 g
Starches: 16.9 g
Protein: 21.5 g
Diabetic Exchanges:
　1 Starch/Bread, 1 Medium-
　Fat Meat, ½ Fat

Cook the pasta according to package directions until al dente, without any added salt or oil.

Meanwhile, heat the margarine and olive oil in a large nonstick skillet over medium heat until margarine melts. Add the shrimp and sauté for 3 minutes, then add the garlic and sauté for 1 minute.

Add the lemon juice, wine, water, salt substitute, and pepper. Simmer for 3 minutes, or until the shrimp are cooked through. Stir in the parsley and toss to coat. Sprinkle the shrimp with the bread crumbs, cover, and simmer for 1 minute.

Divide the pasta among 4 plates and top each with an equal amount of the shrimp and sauce. Garnish each with a wedge of lemon, if desired.

Variations

Chicken can be used instead of shrimp, but make sure the chicken is cooked through before you start the "add lemon juice" step. You can also add items such as fresh-packed sun-dried tomatoes, roasted red peppers, or sliced mushrooms.

Tequila Shrimp

Tequila, a Mexican liquor made from blue agave plants, gets its name from the town it originated in. The tequila called for here imparts a unique flavor without overpowering the dish. This makes a great summer entrée served with rice and a grilled vegetable.

Yield: 4 servings

1 tablespoon light margarine
1 pound large shrimp, peeled and deveined
2 cloves garlic, minced
1 lime, cut into 6 wedges
2 tablespoons tequila, Anejo or Blanco
2 tablespoons water
¼ cup chopped cilantro

Nutritional Information Per Serving (¼ of recipe):

Calories: 126
Fat: 3.1 g
  Saturated Fat: 0.3 g
  Monounsaturated Fat: 0.8 g
  Polyunsaturated Fat: 1.1 g
Cholesterol: 134 mg
Sodium: 151 mg
Carbohydrate: 1.8 g
Dietary Fiber: 0.1 g
Sugars: 1.3 g
Starches: 0 g
Protein: 18 g
Diabetic Exchanges:
  2 Medium-Fat Meat

Melt the margarine in a large nonstick skillet over medium heat. Add the shrimp and sauté until pink and firm to the touch, about 4 minutes. Add the garlic and sauté for 1 minute. Squeeze in the juice of 2 lime wedges, then toss the 2 wedges into the skillet. Add the tequila, water, and cilantro and simmer for 2 minutes, or until the shrimp are cooked. Serve at once, using the remaining lime wedges as garnish.

Garlic Shrimp over Couscous

Shrimp are sautéed with garlic and simmered with sherry, lemon, and fresh parsley before being served over couscous for a flavorful main dish that is easy to prepare. You can substitute a serving of pasta or rice instead of couscous if you prefer.

Yield: 4 servings

**Nutritional Information
Per Serving (¼ of recipe):**

Calories: 185
Fat: 4.3 g
  Saturated Fat: 0.6 g
  Monounsaturated Fat: 2.6 g
  Polyunsaturated Fat: 0.6 g
Cholesterol: 64 mg
Sodium: 69 mg
Carbohydrate: 20.3 g
Dietary Fiber: 1.3 g
Sugars: 0.8 g
Starches: 0.1 g
Protein: 11.8 g
Diabetic Exchanges:
  1½ Starch/Bread,
  1 Medium-Fat Meat

1 tablespoon olive oil
28 medium shrimp (about 1 pound), peeled and
    deveined
¼ teaspoon red pepper flakes
3 garlic cloves, chopped
¼ cup dry sherry
1 tablespoon lemon juice
2 tablespoons minced fresh parsley
Pinch freshly ground black pepper, or to taste
2 cups cooked couscous
4 lemon wedges

Heat a large nonstick skillet over medium heat until hot. Add the oil, shrimp, and red pepper flakes and sauté for 3 minutes. Add the garlic and continue to sauté until the shrimp are pink and firm to the touch. Add the sherry, lemon juice, and parsley and simmer for 2 minutes. Season with black pepper and serve over couscous with lemon wedges.

Shrimp Jambalaya

Our version of the renowned Creole dish lets you combine all the ingredients in a casserole so you can just pop it in the oven. This recipe results in a fairly spicy dish, so adjust the spices according to your taste.

Yield: 4 servings

Nutritional Information Per Serving (¼ of recipe):

Calories: 357
Fat: 9.9 g
  Saturated Fat: 2.7 g
  Monounsaturated Fat: 1.4 g
  Polyunsaturated Fat: 1.4 g
Cholesterol: 193 mg
Sodium: 408 mg
Carbohydrate: 36 g
Dietary Fiber: 2.7 g
Sugars: 4.6 g
Starches: 0.4 g
Protein: 32 g
Diabetic Exchanges:
  1 Starch/Bread, 2 Medium-
  Fat Meat, 5 Vegetable

Canola cooking spray
½ cup Homemade Chicken Broth (page 66) or
    reduced-sodium, low-fat chicken broth
¾ pound medium shrimp, peeled and deveined
2 cups cooked white rice
¼ pound smoked sausage, sliced or chopped
1 14.5-ounce can low-sodium diced tomatoes
¼ cup finely chopped yellow onion
1 clove garlic, minced
½ cup diced green bell pepper
2 teaspoons Creole Seasoning Mix (page 215) or
    No-Salt Cajun Spice Mix (page 215)
½ teaspoon hot pepper sauce

Preheat oven to 375 degrees F. Spray the bottom of a casserole with cooking spray.

Combine all the remaining ingredients in a large bowl and stir until well combined. Pour into the prepared casserole, cover, and bake for 35 minutes, or until the shrimp are cooked.

Scallops au Gratin

You'll find it hard to believe that this rich, creamy dish doesn't contain heavy cream and tons of fat! Serve with brown rice and a cooked vegetable, such as Basil Green Beans (page 155).

Yield: 4 servings

Nutritional Information Per Serving (¼ of recipe):

Calories: 258
Fat: 6.2 g
  Saturated Fat: 2.8 g
  Monounsaturated Fat: 1.8 g
  Polyunsaturated Fat: 0.9 g
Cholesterol: 52 mg
Sodium: 419 mg
Carbohydrate: 15.1 g
Dietary Fiber: 0.6 g
Sugars: 3.2 g
Starches: 1.5 g
Protein: 32.6 g
Diabetic Exchanges:
  2 Medium-Fat Meat,
  1 Fat-Free Milk

Canola cooking spray
2 teaspoons cornstarch
2 tablespoons water
1 teaspoon margarine
⅓ cup finely chopped shallots
1 pound bay scallops, cleaned
¼ teaspoon dried tarragon
2 tablespoons dry white wine
⅓ cup evaporated nonfat milk
1½ teaspoons Dijon mustard
2 tablespoons shredded reduced-fat Jarlsberg cheese
¼ cup dry plain bread crumbs
2 teaspoons grated Romano cheese
⅛ teaspoon black pepper
1 tablespoon chopped fresh parsley, or 1 teaspoon dried parsley flakes

Preheat oven to 400 degrees F.

In a small bowl, combine the cornstarch and water and stir until smooth.

Heat a large nonstick skillet over medium heat. Away from the heat source, spray with the cooking spray. Return to the heat and add the margarine. Add the shallots and sauté for 1 minute. Add the scallops and tarragon and sauté for 4 minutes, or until the scallops become somewhat firm to the touch. Remove the scallops to a bowl and set aside.

To the same skillet, add the white wine, evaporated milk, and mustard and bring to a simmer. Slowly stir in the cornstarch mixture and continue to cook until thickened, about 1 minute. Remove the skillet from the heat and stir in the Jarlsberg cheese until it melts. Return the scallops to the skillet and stir so that they are well coated.

Combine the bread crumbs, Romano cheese, and black pepper in a small bowl.

Divide the scallop mixture evenly among 4 1-cup oven-proof au gratin dishes, or pour the entire mixture into a 1-quart oven-proof dish. Sprinkle with the bread crumb mixture and spray lightly with cooking spray. Bake for 12 to 15 minutes, or until the crumbs turn golden and the liquid bubbles.

To serve, place each individual au gratin dish on a dinner plate and sprinkle with parsley. If you used one large baking dish, divide the scallops among 4 dinner plates and top each with parsley.

Linguine with Herbed Porcini Clam Sauce

Whole baby clams, garlic, and porcini mushrooms are sautéed with Italian seasoning and tossed with linguine for a simple-to-prepare gourmet meal. Fresh porcini mushrooms can be difficult to find in supermarkets, mainly because of their cost and relatively short shelf life. Dried porcini are readily available and work quite well in dishes such as this one.

Yield: 4 servings

1 pound linguine
Canola cooking spray
½ teaspoon olive oil
⅔ cup chopped yellow onion
1 to 2 cloves garlic, minced
1½ cups sliced fresh porcini mushrooms, or 1½ to 2 ounces dried porcini mushrooms, reconstituted
⅓ cup dry white wine
2 tablespoons chopped fresh parsley
1 teaspoon no-salt Italian seasoning
¼ teaspoon freshly ground black pepper
1 16-ounce can whole baby clams, chopped, reserve 2 tablespoons clam juice
Chopped fresh parsley, optional garnish

Nutritional Information Per Serving (¼ of recipe):

Calories: 323
Fat: 2.8 g
  Saturated Fat: 0.2 g
  Monounsaturated Fat: 0.7 g
  Polyunsaturated Fat: 0.9 g
Cholesterol: 48 mg
Sodium: 86 mg
Carbohydrate: 44 g
Dietary Fiber: 2.3 g
Sugars: 2.1 g
Starches: 33.9 g
Protein: 25.2 g
Diabetic Exchanges:
  3 Starch/Bread, 1 Medium-Fat Meat

Cook the linguine according to package directions until al dente, without any added salt or oil.

Heat a large nonstick skillet over medium heat. Away from the heat source, spray with cooking spray and add the oil. Sauté the onion until softened, about 5 minutes. Add the garlic and mushrooms and sauté for 3 minutes. Add the wine, parsley, Italian seasoning, and black pepper and cook for 2 minutes. Stir in the clams and the reserved clam juice and continue to cook for 2 to 3 minutes. Add the cooked pasta and toss until well coated. Divide among 4 plates and serve immediately. Garnish with chopped fresh parsley, if desired.

Baked Sole Dijon

The classic French flavors of Dijon mustard and thyme are combined with nonfat yogurt and used to coat sole fillets, which are then baked until flaky and moist. Steamed asparagus (or green beans) and rice are excellent accompaniments.

Canola cooking spray
½ cup plain nonfat yogurt
1 tablespoon Dijon mustard
½ teaspoon dried thyme
1 teaspoon lemon juice
4 4-ounce sole fillets

Preheat oven to 375 degrees F. Spray a large baking dish with cooking spray.

In a medium bowl, combine yogurt, mustard, thyme, and lemon juice. Dip each fillet into the Dijon-yogurt marinade until well coated and place in the prepared baking dish. Spoon remaining sauce over the fillets and spread evenly. Bake for 10 to 12 minutes, or until the fish flakes easily with a fork.

Yield: 4 servings

Nutritional Information Per Serving (¼ of recipe):
Calories: 152
Fat: 1.9 g
　Saturated Fat: 0.4 g
　Monounsaturated Fat: 0.3 g
　Polyunsaturated Fat: 0.7 g
Cholesterol: 78 mg
Sodium: 233 mg
Carbohydrate: 2.7 g
Dietary Fiber: 0 g
Sugars: 2.6 g
Starches: 0 g
Protein: 29.4 g
Diabetic Exchanges: 4 Very
　Lean Meat

Halibut Topped with Vidalia Onion and Raspberry-Balsamic Sauce

Grilled halibut is topped with a sweet and fruity balsamic sauce reduced with sautéed Vidalia onion. Vidalia onions, the official state vegetable of Georgia, contain more water and sugar than most other types of onion and are a bit more perishable. Refrigerate them if you want to have them on hand for an extended period of time.

Yield: 4 servings

Nutritional Information Per Serving (¼ of recipe):

Calories: 199
Fat: 4 g
  Saturated Fat: 0.2 g
  Monounsaturated Fat: 1.9 g
  Polyunsaturated Fat: 1.2 g
Cholesterol: 42 mg
Sodium: 74 mg
Carbohydrate: 12.3 g
Dietary Fiber: 1 g
Sugars: 9.1 g
Starches: 2.2 g
Protein: 27.2 g
Diabetic Exchanges:
  2 Medium-Fat Meat, 1 Fruit

Canola cooking spray
1 teaspoon olive oil
1 large Vidalia onion, or sweet yellow onion, thinly sliced
½ cup Homemade Vegetable Broth (page 68) or reduced-sodium, low-fat vegetable broth
2 tablespoons water
2 tablespoons red raspberry spreadable fruit
¼ cup balsamic vinegar
4 3½-ounce halibut fillets

Heat a nonstick skillet over medium heat. Away from the heat source, spray with cooking spray. Return to the heat and add oil. Sauté the onion for 10 minutes, or until soft and golden. Add the broth and water and simmer for 5 minutes. Stir in the raspberry spreadable fruit and vinegar and simmer for 2 minutes; set aside.

Meanwhile, heat a grill or grill pan over medium-high heat. Lightly oil the grill rack with canola oil using a paper towel or, away from the heat source, spray the grill pan with cooking spray. Grill the halibut until cooked through, 3 to 4 minutes per side. Serve with warm Vidalia sauce spooned over each piece of grilled halibut.

Orange Roughy with Sun-Dried Tomato Tapenade

Tapenade, which originated in France, is traditionally a thick paste made from anchovies, olives, capers, olive oil, and various seasonings. It is often spread on crostini for canapés or served alongside crudite or certain seafood dishes. In addition to the traditional components of tapenade, this dish also uses sweet sun-dried tomatoes to richly flavor the flaky, moist orange roughy.

Yield: 2 servings, can be doubled

Nutritional Information Per Serving (½ of recipe):
Calories: 138
Fat: 2.6 g
  Saturated Fat: 0.2 g
  Monounsaturated Fat: 1.4 g
  Polyunsaturated Fat: 0.3 g
Cholesterol: 26 mg
Sodium: 765 mg
Carbohydrate: 8.5 g
Dietary Fiber: 2 g
Sugars: 0.4 g
Starches: 0 g
Protein: 19.6 g
Diabetic Exchanges:
  1 Medium-Fat Meat,
  2 Vegetable

Canola cooking spray
2 4-ounce orange roughy fillets, rinsed
¼ cup water
1 tablespoon dry white wine
½ cup chopped sun-dried tomatoes, fresh-packed
  (not in oil)
⅛ teaspoon dried thyme
⅛ teaspoon dried sweet basil
Pinch ground black pepper
2 tablespoons sliced black olives
1 tablespoon chopped capers
1 anchovy fillet, chopped
1 clove garlic, chopped
Lemon slices, optional

Preheat oven to 375 degrees F.

Spray the bottom of a casserole with cooking spray. Place the fish fillets in a single layer in the casserole. Combine the remaining ingredients in a bowl and spoon over the fish. Cover the casserole and bake for 25 to 30 minutes, or until the fish flakes easily with a fork. Remove the fillets to 2 dinner plates and spoon the tapenade over and around it. Garnish with lemon slices, if desired.

Steak au Poivre

Tenderloin is coated with three types of peppercorns, along with fennel, then pan-broiled and topped with a rich brandy cream sauce. Serve with steamed green beans or asparagus.

2 teaspoons whole black peppercorns
½ teaspoon whole white peppercorns
½ teaspoon dried green peppercorns
1 teaspoon fennel seeds, or ¼ teaspoon ground fennel
4 4-ounce tenderloin steaks, well trimmed
1 teaspoon olive oil
1 cup Homemade Beef Broth (page 67) or canned reduced-sodium, low-fat beef broth
6 tablespoons evaporated nonfat milk
2 tablespoons brandy or Cognac

Yield: 4 servings

**Nutritional Information
Per Serving (¼ of recipe):**

Calories: 333
Fat: 15.6 g
  Saturated Fat: 5.7 g
  Monounsaturated Fat: 6.6 g
  Polyunsaturated Fat: 0.7 g
Cholesterol: 99 mg
Sodium: 107 mg
Carbohydrate: 4.3 g
Dietary Fiber: 0.6 g
Sugars: 0.1 g
Starches: 0 g
Protein: 33.8 g
Diabetic Exchanges:
  4 Medium-Fat Meat

In a resealable plastic bag, crush the peppercorns and fennel seeds until coarse using a kitchen mallet. Pat the steaks dry and coat evenly with peppercorn-fennel mixture, pressing it into both sides (you don't need to use all of the peppercorn mixture).

Heat a large heavy skillet over medium-high heat until hot. Add the oil and swirl so it coats the bottom of the pan.

Place the seasoned steaks in the hot skillet and pan-broil until the meat is medium-rare, about 3 to 4 minutes per side (or cooked to your liking). Transfer the steaks to individual dinner plates.

Reduce skillet heat to medium. Add the beef broth and scrape up any remaining browned bits left in the skillet. Stir in the evaporated milk and brandy and continue to simmer until the sauce thickens, 1 to 2 minutes. Spoon equal amounts of the sauce over the cooked steaks and serve.

Salisbury Steak with Mushroom Gravy

Salisbury steak is named after a nineteenth-century nutritionist, J.H. Salisbury. Our version mimics the classic recipe that combines ground beef with bread crumbs, egg, onion, and spices, and even includes a savory mushroom gravy to top it. Serve with our Mock Mashed Potatoes (page 169) for a savory down-home meal without all of the carbohydrate and fat you would expect.

Yield: 4 servings

Nutritional Information
Per Serving (¼ of recipe):

Calories: 269
Fat: 7.4 g
  Saturated Fat: 3 g
  Monounsaturated Fat: 2.7 g
  Polyunsaturated Fat: 0.6 g
Cholesterol: 81 mg
Sodium: 163 mg
Carbohydrate: 12.3 g
Dietary Fiber: 1.7 g
Sugars: 0.3 g
Starches: 0 g
Protein: 39 g
Diabetic Exchanges:
  5 Lean Meat

Canola cooking spray
½ teaspoon canola oil
2 tablespoons finely chopped yellow onion
1 teaspoon minced garlic
½ cup finely chopped white mushrooms
1 teaspoon Worcestershire sauce
1 teaspoon dried parsley flakes
⅛ teaspoon ground black pepper
1 pound 95% lean ground beef
2 tablespoons unseasoned bread crumbs
1 egg white
1 recipe Savory Mushroom Gravy (page 208)

Preheat oven to 375 degrees F.

Heat a small nonstick skillet over medium-low heat. Away from the heat source, spray with cooking spray. Return to the heat and add the canola oil and onion. Sauté for 5 minutes, or until softened. Add the garlic and sauté for 1 minute. Remove the onion and garlic to a large mixing bowl.

Add the chopped mushrooms, Worcestershire sauce, parsley, and black pepper. Add the ground beef, bread crumbs, and egg white. Break up the beef and mix until very well combined.

Form the beef mixture into four equal-sized balls. Flatten each ball into a ⅓-inch-thick oval patty. Place the patties in a baking dish sprayed with cooking spray and bake for 30 minutes, or until browned, firm to touch, and cooked through.

Meanwhile, prepare the Savory Mushroom Gravy.

Serve each Salisbury steak topped with an equal amount of gravy.

Rustic Pot Roast with Vegetables

By using a lean cut of beef and limited oil, we were able to create a pot roast dinner that can fit into just about anyone's meal plan. Herbes de Provence is a spice blend that can be found in the spice section of most supermarkets. For a pot roast with a stronger tomato base, stir in one 8-ounce can of tomato paste when you add the tomato sauce.

½ cup all-purpose flour
½ teaspoon ground black pepper
3 pounds eye of round beef roast, select cut, fat trimmed
Canola cooking spray
3 medium cloves garlic
1 cup sliced yellow onion
2 cups sliced carrots
4 cups Homemade Beef Broth (page 67) or reduced-sodium, low-fat beef broth
1 16-ounce can reduced-sodium or no-salt-added tomato sauce
1 cup Burgundy or other dry red wine
¾ cup water
1 teaspoon Herbes de Provence
1 bay leaf
½ pound baby turnips, peeled
½ pound baby parsnips, peeled
2 teaspoons chopped fresh parsley

Yield: 12 servings

Nutritional Information Per Serving (¹⁄₁₂ of recipe):

Calories: 222
Fat: 4 g
 Saturated Fat: 1.4 g
 Monounsaturated Fat: 1.7 g
 Polyunsaturated Fat: 0.2 g
Cholesterol: 61 mg
Sodium: 94 mg
Carbohydrate: 14.6 g
Dietary Fiber: 2.4 g
Sugars: 2.5 g
Starches: 1.9 g
Protein: 27.5 g
Diabetic Exchanges:
 3 Medium-Fat Meat,
 4 Vegetable

In a large mixing bowl, combine the flour and pepper. Dredge the beef roast in the flour mix until lightly coated.

Heat a large heavy stockpot over medium-high heat. Away from the heat source, coat the bottom with cooking spray. Return to the heat and brown the beef on all sides. Set the beef aside on a large plate.

Add the garlic, onion, and carrots to the pot and sauté for 3 minutes. Stir in the broth, tomato sauce, wine, water, Herbes de Provence, and bay leaf. Return the roast to the pan, along with any juices that collected on the plate. Add the turnips and parsnips and bring to a boil. Cover and reduce heat to low. Simmer for 2 to 2½ hours, or until roast is fork tender.

Transfer the roast to a large serving platter. Discard the bay leaf and spoon the vegetables around the roast. Spoon the sauce over the roast and sprinkle with fresh parsley.

Tex-Mex Casserole

Tex-Mex, a style of cooking that incorporates both Mexican and Texas-style cookery, includes dishes such as chili, nachos, and burritos. This casserole offers a creamy, meaty-tasting, and somewhat spicy dish that is super for lunch or dinner.

8 ounces elbow macaroni
1 cup chopped, seeded tomato
1 teaspoon canola oil
1/3 cup chopped yellow onion
1 cup sliced white mushrooms
1 clove garlic, minced
2 tablespoons minced pickled jalapeño pepper
3 ounces 95% lean ground beef
1 tablespoon all-purpose flour
1/4 cup skim milk
1 cup evaporated nonfat milk, divided
2 tablespoons light sour cream
5 ounces shredded reduced-fat, reduced-sodium sharp Cheddar cheese
1/2 teaspoon hot pepper sauce
1/8 teaspoon ground black pepper

Yield: 4 servings

**Nutritional Information
Per Serving (1/4 of recipe):**

Calories: 208
Fat: 5 g
  Saturated Fat: 2.7 g
  Monounsaturated Fat: 1.5 g
  Polyunsaturated Fat: 0.4 g
Cholesterol: 25 mg
Sodium: 33 mg
Carbohydrate: 21.8 g
Dietary Fiber: 1.7 g
Sugars: 1.1 g
Starches: 12.7 g
Protein: 18.9 g
Diabetic Exchanges:
  1 Starch/Bread, 2 Lean Meat,
  1 Vegetable

Cook the pasta according to package directions until al dente, without any added salt or oil. Drain and return to the pot you cooked it in. Stir in the chopped tomato and set aside.

While the pasta is cooking, heat the oil over medium heat in a medium nonstick skillet. Add the onion and mushrooms and sauté until the onion becomes golden and the mushrooms soften, about 10 minutes. Add the garlic and jalapeño pepper and sauté for 2 minutes.

Cook the ground beef in a small nonstick skillet over medium heat. Use a wooden spoon to break the beef up into little bits as it cooks. Once the meat is cooked, transfer it to the pot with the pasta. Stir in the sautéed vegetables.

In a small bowl, stir the flour and skim milk until smooth. In a small saucepan, heat ¾ cup evaporated nonfat milk and the sour cream over medium-high heat. Once it begins to bubble, whisk in the flour mixture. Reduce heat to medium and continue to whisk until mixture begins to thicken, about 2 minutes. Stir in the shredded cheese and continue to stir until the cheese melts. Whisk in the remaining ¼ cup evaporated milk, hot sauce, and black pepper.

Add the cheese sauce to the cooked pasta, beef, and vegetables and stir well. Transfer to a baking dish or casserole and broil until the top has crisped but not burned. Divide equally among 4 plates and serve hot.

Classic Italian Meatballs in Pomodoro Sauce

These meatballs really are a classic. Once cooked and cooled, you can freeze them for at least a month in a sealed freezer bag or container and then thaw in the microwave or overnight in the refrigerator. Make sure you chop the onion finely; otherwise the meatballs may break apart. For classic pasta with meatballs, serve 2 meatballs over ½ cup penne with ¼ cup sauce and sprinkle with grated Parmesan or Romano cheese.

Yield: About 16 meatballs, or 8 servings

Nutritional Information Per Serving (2 meatballs and ¼ cup sauce):

Calories: 159
Fat: 3.7 g
  Saturated Fat: 1.5 g
  Monounsaturated Fat: 1.4 g
  Polyunsaturated Fat: 0.3 g
Cholesterol: 39 mg
Sodium: 133 mg
Carbohydrate: 12.9 g
Dietary Fiber: 1.6 g
Sugars: 0.3 g
Starches: 0 g
Protein: 18.9 g
Diabetic Exchanges:
  1 Medium-Fat Meat,
  3 Vegetable

Canola cooking spray
1 pound 95% lean ground beef
1 clove garlic, minced
3 tablespoons very finely chopped yellow onion
2 tablespoons dried parsley flakes, or 3 tablespoons minced fresh parsley
¼ teaspoon no-salt Italian seasoning
¾ cup unseasoned bread crumbs
Rocco's Pomodoro Sauce (page 207)

Preheat oven to 375 degrees F. Coat a nonstick baking sheet or roasting pan with cooking spray and set aside.

In a large mixing bowl, break up the ground beef into little bits with a spoon. Add the garlic, onion, parsley, Italian seasoning, and bread crumbs and mix together thoroughly. Crumble the beef between your fingers with the other ingredients. The more broken up the meat is, the more flavorful and tender the meatballs will be.

Shape the meat mixture into 1½-ounce balls and place on the baking sheet spaced so they are not touching. Bake for 25 to 30 minutes, or until browned and cooked through.

Meanwhile, prepare Rocco's Pomodoro Sauce.

When the meatballs are done, put them in a saucepan with Rocco's Pomodoro Sauce and simmer over medium-low heat for 5 to 10 minutes, stirring occasionally. Serve meatballs with ¼ cup of sauce.

Veal Piccata

Veal is sautéed until tender and tossed with a lemon-caper sauce in this version of one of the most popular dishes on restaurant menus. Surprisingly easy to make for a family dinner or a dinner party, it is much lower in fat and calories than the restaurant version. You can make this dish using chicken breast or pork loin if you prefer, but make sure the meat is cooked thoroughly before serving. Serve with no-cholesterol egg noodles or brown rice and steamed broccoli or asparagus for a well-rounded meal.

Yield: 4 servings

Nutritional Information Per Serving (¼ of recipe):

Calories: 263
Fat: 5.5 g
  Saturated Fat: 1.6 g
  Monounsaturated Fat: 2 g
  Polyunsaturated Fat: 0.9 g
Cholesterol: 114 mg
Sodium: 192 mg
Carbohydrate: 11.1 g
Dietary Fiber: 0.8 g
Sugars: 0.4 g
Starches: 0.5 g
Protein: 32.7 g
Diabetic Exchanges:
  3 Medium-Fat Meat

4 3-ounce veal cutlets, fat trimmed
⅓ cup all-purpose flour
Canola cooking spray
1 teaspoon canola oil
¼ cup Homemade Chicken Broth (page 66) or
    reduced-sodium, low-fat chicken broth
½ cup dry sherry or dry white wine
¼ cup lemon juice
2 tablespoons capers, rinsed and drained
1 tablespoon chopped fresh parsley, or ¾ teaspoon
    dried parsley flakes
4 lemon slices

Pound the veal cutlets to a thickness of ¼ inch. Dredge the cutlets in flour until lightly coated.

Shake off the excess and discard the remaining flour.

Heat a large nonstick skillet over medium-high heat. Away from the heat source, spray with cooking spray. Return to the heat and add the oil. Add the veal cutlets and sauté until golden, about 2 minutes per side. Remove the veal to a plate and keep warm.

To the same skillet, add the broth, sherry, lemon juice, and capers. Cook over medium-high heat, stirring, until sauce is reduced by one-third. Reduce heat to medium and add the cutlets along with any juices that collected on the plate. Heat for 2 minutes, then transfer to a serving platter. Sprinkle with parsley and top with lemon slices to serve.

Mediterranean Grilled Lamb Chops

Lamb chops are heavily seasoned with a Mediterranean-style rub and grilled, resulting in a robust dish perfect for a summertime dinner. You can also use the same rub on poultry or beef prior to grilling or broiling. Serve with Grilled Vegetables (page 161) and Roasted Herbed Potatoes (page 169), if desired.

Yield: 2 servings, can be doubled

2 tablespoons olive oil
1 tablespoon minced shallot
1 tablespoon minced garlic
2 tablespoons chopped fresh parsley, or 1 teaspoon dried parsley flakes
⅛ teaspoon dried oregano
⅛ teaspoon dried thyme
⅛ teaspoon dried marjoram
Ground black pepper
4 4-ounce loin lamb chops
Canola cooking spray

Nutritional Information Per Serving (1 chop):
Calories: 149
Fat: 8.3 g
  Saturated Fat: 2.2 g
  Monounsaturated Fat: 4.6 g
  Polyunsaturated Fat: 0.6 g
Cholesterol: 48 mg
Sodium: 46 mg
Carbohydrate: 2.6 g
Dietary Fiber: 0.4 g
Sugars: 1.5 g
Starches: 0.6 g
Protein: 15.6 g
Diabetic Exchanges:
  2 Medium-Fat Meat

Combine the oil, shallot, garlic, herbs, and black pepper in a small bowl.

On a large plate, press the rub into both sides of the chops.

Heat a grill pan to medium-high heat (or heat a gas or charcoal grill). Away from the heat source, coat the pan with cooking spray. Return the pan to the heat, and grill the chops until cooked through, about 3 to 4 minutes per side.

Greek Gyros with Tzatziki Sauce

A gyro is a classic Greek sandwich consisting of roasted lamb that is sliced and served wrapped in a pita with onions, peppers, and yogurt-cucumber sauce. In our version, ground lamb is marinated in a blend of herbs and spices, grilled, and then served in a pita with onion, lettuce, tomatoes, and our own Tzatziki Sauce. Similar to our Chicken Souvlaki Plate (page 102), this is great for lunch.

For the Marinade:
2 tablespoons olive oil
¼ cup lemon juice
2 cloves garlic, minced
½ teaspoon dried thyme
½ teaspoon dried oregano
⅛ teaspoon freshly ground black pepper

For the Meat Mix:
¾ pound lean ground lamb
1 teaspoon minced garlic
¼ teaspoon dried oregano
¼ teaspoon ground cumin
⅛ teaspoon dried thyme
¼ teaspoon dried parsley flakes
⅛ teaspoon freshly ground black pepper

Remaining Ingredients:
4 tablespoons Tzatziki Sauce (page 210)
Canola cooking spray
2 fat-free pita pockets
2 vine-ripened tomatoes, thinly sliced
1 cup iceberg lettuce leaves, torn into bite-size pieces
1 yellow or red onion, thinly sliced

Whisk all marinade ingredients in a bowl and set aside.

Yield: 4 servings, 1 gyro per serving

Nutritional Information Per Serving (1 gyro):

Calories: 351
Fat: 7.6 g
  Saturated Fat: 3.2 g
  Monounsaturated Fat: 3.2 g
  Polyunsaturated Fat: 0.3 g
Cholesterol: 80 mg
Sodium: 401 mg
Carbohydrate: 33.1 g
Dietary Fiber: 2.1 g
Sugars: 6.8 g
Starches: 0.6 g
Protein: 39 g
Diabetic Exchanges:
  3 Starch/Bread, 3 Lean Meat, 4 Vegetable

Combine all meat mix ingredients in a large bowl and mix well. Shape the meat into 3-ounce meatballs and flatten into ½-inch-thick patties. Arrange the patties on a plate in one layer and pour the marinade over the meat. Flip the patties every 5 minutes for 25 minutes to evenly coat.

Prepare the Tzatziki Sauce.

Heat a grill or grill pan over medium heat. Spray with cooking spray away from the heat. Return to the heat and grill lamb patties for 3 to 4 minutes per side, or until cooked to the degree of doneness you prefer.

Slice each pita in half and open the pita pocket. Stuff each half with sliced tomato, lettuce, onion, and 1 tablespoon Tzatziki Sauce. Slice each cooked lamb patty into ½-inch-wide slices and stuff into the pita. Serve immediately.

Apricot Grilled Pork Tenderloin

This is an excellent dish for a barbecue or outdoor party. Pork tenderloin is marinated with a simple orange-apricot sauce right in the middle of the cooking process, resulting in a sweet and slightly crunchy outside and a moist, juicy inside. Tenderloin is the leanest cut of pork, with a 3-ounce portion containing about 140 calories and 4 grams of fat, which is comparable to chicken breast.

Yield: 4 servings

Nutritional Information Per Serving (¼ of recipe):

Calories: 202
Fat: 4.1 g
  Saturated Fat: 1.5 g
  Monounsaturated Fat: 1.5 g
  Polyunsaturated Fat: 0.3 g
Cholesterol: 65 mg
Sodium: 55 mg
Carbohydrate: 16.6 g
Dietary Fiber: 0.3 g
Sugars: 13.6 g
Starches: 2.7 g
Protein: 23.8 g
Diabetic Exchanges:
  2 Medium-Fat Meat, 2 Fruit

¼ cup apricot spreadable fruit
¼ cup orange juice, no-pulp style
Dash ground black pepper
1 1-pound pork tenderloin

In a large mixing bowl, combine the spreadable fruit, orange juice, and black pepper.

Heat an outdoor grill to medium heat and grill the pork for about 13 minutes. Remove and soak in the apricot marinade for 5 minutes, turning often.

Return the meat to the grill for another 2 minutes, then soak in the apricot marinade for 2 minutes. Grill for another 3 minutes, or until fully cooked, discarding all of the remaining marinade. Slice the pork and serve.

Italian Roast Pork

Pork loin is rubbed with a mixture of dried herbs and spices and roasted, resulting in a flavorful crust on the outside and a moist, juicy inside. Slice into 3- to 4-ounce portions and serve with rice and fresh vegetables, if desired.

Yield: 6 to 8 servings

Canola cooking spray
½ teaspoon garlic powder
¼ teaspoon crushed red pepper flakes
¼ teaspoon ground black pepper
2 teaspoons no-salt Italian seasoning
1 2-pound boneless top loin pork roast

Preheat oven to 375 degrees F. Coat a roasting pan with cooking spray.

Combine all the seasonings in a small bowl. Coat the pork loin with the mixed seasonings and place in the prepared roasting pan. Roast for 50 minutes, or until cooked thoroughly. Remove from oven and allow to stand for 5 minutes before slicing.

Nutritional Information Per Serving (⅙ of recipe):

Calories: 139
Fat: 4.9 g
  Saturated Fat: 1.7 g
  Monounsaturated Fat: 2.1 g
  Polyunsaturated Fat: 0.7 g
Cholesterol: 62 mg
Sodium: 66 mg
Carbohydrate: 0.1 g
Dietary Fiber: 0 g
Sugars: 0 g
Starches: 0 g
Protein: 21.5 g
Diabetic Exchanges:
  2 Medium-Fat Meat

Spinach Mushroom Lasagne

Spinach and mushrooms are layered between lasagna noodles along with a combination of cheeses, herbs, and Nona's Italian Marinara Sauce (page 205) to make a lasagne that nobody will believe has only 5 grams of fat per serving.

Yield: 8 servings

**Nutritional Information
Per Serving (⅛ of recipe):**

Calories: 224
Fat: 5 g
  Saturated Fat: 3 g
  Monounsaturated Fat: 1.5 g
  Polyunsaturated Fat: 0.4 g
Cholesterol: 27 mg
Sodium: 197 mg
Carbohydrate: 31.2 g
Dietary Fiber: 3.8 g
Sugars: 5.2 g
Starches: 17.6 g
Protein: 16.4 g
Diabetic Exchanges:
  1 Starch/Bread, 4 Vegetable,
  1 Fat

9 lasagna noodles, uncooked
1 teaspoon olive oil
1 cup chopped yellow onion
1 clove garlic, minced
1 tablespoon chopped fresh basil, or ½ teaspoon
  dried basil
½ teaspoon dried oregano
2 cups thinly sliced white mushrooms
¼ cup chopped fresh parsley
Pinch of freshly ground black pepper, or to taste
⅛ teaspoon crushed red pepper flakes
1 10-ounce package frozen spinach, thawed,
  drained, and squeezed dry
2 cups Nona's Italian Marinara Sauce (page 205) or
  reduced-sodium, low-fat marinara sauce
1 15-ounce container part-skim ricotta cheese
¾ cup shredded part-skim mozzarella cheese
Grated Romano cheese, optional

Cook the pasta according to package directions until al dente, without any added oil or salt. Drain and rinse under cold water until cool enough to handle.

Meanwhile, heat the olive oil over medium heat in a medium nonstick skillet. Add the onion and sauté for 5 minutes, or until softened. Add the garlic, basil, and oregano and sauté for 1 minute. Remove the onion mixture to a bowl and set aside.

To the same skillet, add the mushrooms and sauté until tender and browned, 5 to 7 minutes. Stir in the parsley, black pepper, crushed red pepper flakes, and half of the onion and garlic mixture. Heat for 1 minute, stirring. Transfer to a bowl and set aside.

Add the spinach to the remaining garlic and onion mixture and set aside.

Preheat oven to 350 degrees F.

Spread ¾ cup marinara sauce over the bottom of a 13-by-9-by-3-inch casserole or lasagna pan. Arrange a layer of 3 lasagna noodles, evenly topped with the spinach mixture, half the ricotta cheese, and ¼ cup mozzarella.

Arrange a second layer of 3 noodles and evenly top with the mushroom mixture, the remaining ricotta cheese, and ¼ cup mozzarella.

Arrange 3 noodles for the top layer. Cover with the remaining marinara sauce and sprinkle with the remaining mozzarella. Bake for 30 minutes, or until heated through and just bubbly on top. Cut into 8 portions and serve with Romano cheese, if desired.

Macaroni and Cheese

Now this is what you call comfort food! Good ol' mac 'n' cheese. In a real hurry? Skip the oven step and just finish it after adding the cooked pasta to the saucepan by heating it, over medium heat, until thickened to the consistency you want. Stir in 1 cup of thawed frozen chopped broccoli right before you put it in the oven for a nice variation (adds minimal calories or carbohydrate and counts as ½ vegetable exchange).

Yield: 4 servings

Nutritional Information Per Serving (¼ of recipe):

Calories: 196
Fat: 3 g
  Saturated Fat: 1.6 g
  Monounsaturated Fat: 0.8 g
  Polyunsaturated Fat: 0.2 g
Cholesterol: 8 mg
Sodium: 92 mg
Carbohydrate: 24.9 g
Dietary Fiber: 0.7 g
Sugars: 6.7 g
Starches: 14.9 g
Protein: 16.3 g
Diabetic Exchanges:
  ½ Starch/Bread, 2 Fat-Free Milk

8 ounces elbow macaroni, uncooked
1 tablespoon all-purpose flour
¼ cup skim milk plus 1 tablespoon, divided
¾ cup evaporated nonfat milk plus 2 tablespoons, divided
1 tablespoon fat-free sour cream
5 ounces shredded reduced-fat, reduced-sodium mild or sharp Cheddar cheese
⅛ teaspoon ground black pepper, or to taste
1 teaspoon grated Romano cheese, optional

Cook the pasta according to package directions until al dente, without any added salt or oil.

Preheat broiler.

In a small bowl, stir the flour into ¼ cup skim milk until smooth.

In a medium saucepan, heat ¾ cup evaporated

milk and the sour cream over medium-high heat until hot, whisking. Whisk in the flour mixture and continue to whisk until the sauce begins to thicken, about 2 minutes.

Reduce heat to medium and whisk in the Cheddar cheese. Continue to whisk until the cheese melts and the sauce is smooth. Whisk in 1 tablespoon skim milk and 2 tablespoons evaporated milk. Stir the pasta and black pepper into the sauce. Heat for 1 minute, stirring, then pour into a 2-quart baking dish or casserole.

Broil until the top forms a crust, 3 to 5 minutes. Serve hot, sprinkled with Romano cheese, if desired.

Greek-Style Orzo with Spinach and Tomatoes

The classic Greek combination of spinach and feta is teamed with lemon, orzo, and Mediterranean seasonings for a filling vegetarian main dish. Orzo, a type of pasta that resembles short-grain rice, works well in soups, salads, and as part of a side or main dish.

1 pound fresh spinach, washed, stems removed, and chopped
16 cherry tomatoes, halved
1 clove garlic, minced
1 tablespoon grated lemon zest
1/4 teaspoon dried oregano
1/8 teaspoon dried basil
2/3 cup orzo, uncooked
1 teaspoon olive oil
2 tablespoons crumbled feta cheese
Freshly ground black pepper, to taste

In a large bowl, combine the spinach, tomatoes, garlic, lemon zest, oregano, and basil.

Cook the orzo according to package directions until al dente, without added salt or oil.

Drain and immediately add to the spinach mixture while the orzo is still hot. Add the olive oil, feta cheese, and black pepper and toss very well.

Yield: 4 servings

Nutritional Information Per Serving (1/4 of recipe):

Calories: 162
Fat: 3.1 g
 Saturated Fat: 0.9 g
 Monounsaturated Fat: 1.1 g
 Polyunsaturated Fat: 0.5 g
Cholesterol: 4 mg
Sodium: 126 mg
Carbohydrate: 27.6 g
Dietary Fiber: 4.2 g
Sugars: 1.5 g
Starches: 19.1 g
Protein: 7.4 g
Diabetic Exchanges:
 2 Starch/Bread

Penne à la Vodka

Penne is coated with a thick and creamy low-fat tomato sauce that has an interesting sharpness courtesy of the vodka (you can omit the vodka, if desired). You can also make this dish with leftover pasta, such as ziti or rigatoni.

1 cup penne pasta, uncooked
¼ cup Homemade Chicken Broth (page 66) or reduced-sodium, low-fat chicken broth
⅔ cup water
¼ cup tomato paste
Pinch salt substitute
Pinch ground black pepper
½ cup evaporated nonfat milk
1 tablespoon vodka
Grated Romano cheese, optional

Cook the pasta according to the package directions until al dente, without added salt or oil. Drain.

Heat the broth and water in a 2-quart saucepan until it begins to boil. Reduce heat to medium and stir in the tomato paste until smooth. Season lightly with salt substitute and pepper and add the evaporated milk. Simmer for 2 minutes, stirring often. Add the vodka and simmer for 1 minute. Add the pasta and heat, stirring, until the sauce coats the pasta.

Divide between 2 dinner plates and sprinkle each serving with ½ teaspoon grated Romano cheese, if desired.

Yield: 2 servings, can be doubled

Nutritional Information Per Serving (½ of recipe):

Calories: 264
Fat: 1.3 g
  Saturated Fat: 0.1 g
  Monounsaturated Fat: 0.2 g
  Polyunsaturated Fat: 0.5 g
Cholesterol: 0 mg
Sodium: 173 mg
Carbohydrate: 47.1 g
Dietary Fiber: 3 g
Sugars: 8.8 g
Starches: 35.1 g
Protein: 12.1 g
Diabetic Exchanges:
  2½ Starch/Bread, ½ Fat-Free Milk

Stuffed Cabbage Rolls

A comfort-food favorite of many families, our version is savory and satisfying without all the fat and sodium you might find in other recipes. You can also use smaller cabbage leaves with ¼ cup of filling in each roll (for a two-roll serving).

Canola cooking spray
3 cups chopped white mushrooms
6 large cabbage leaves
¾ pound 95% or 97% lean ground beef
1 cup cooked brown rice
1 egg white
½ cup chopped yellow onion
1 clove garlic, minced
1 teaspoon no-salt Italian seasoning
⅛ teaspoon ground black pepper

For the Sauce:
1 16-ounce can reduced-sodium or no-salt-added tomato sauce
1 teaspoon no-salt Italian seasoning
⅛ teaspoon crushed red pepper flakes, or more to taste
¼ teaspoon ground black pepper
¼ teaspoon garlic powder

Yield: 6 servings, can be doubled

Nutritional Information Per Serving (⅙ of recipe):

Calories: 176
Fat: 3.6 g
  Saturated Fat: 1.4 g
  Monounsaturated Fat: 1.3 g
  Polyunsaturated Fat: 0.4 g
Cholesterol: 39 mg
Sodium: 71 mg
Carbohydrate: 16.1 g
Dietary Fiber: 2.6 g
Sugars: 3.6 g
Starches: 6.6 g
Protein: 20.3 g
Diabetic Exchanges:
  ½ Starch/Bread, 2 Lean
  Meat, 1 Vegetable

Heat a nonstick skillet over medium-high heat. Away from the heat source, spray with cooking spray. Return to the heat and sauté the mushrooms until tender. Set aside to cool.

Cook the cabbage leaves in boiling water until wilted, about 1 minute. Drain and rinse under cold water.

Preheat oven to 350 degrees F.

In a large bowl, combine the mushrooms, ground beef, rice, egg white, onion, garlic, Italian seasoning, and black pepper and mix well.

Lay the cabbage leaves out flat and divide the meat mixture evenly among them. Fold the ends of each leaf over and roll up (like a burrito). Place the cabbage rolls, seam side down, in a single layer in a casserole or baking dish just large enough to fit all of the rolls.

To make the sauce: Combine the tomato sauce, Italian seasoning, red pepper flakes, black pepper, and garlic powder. Spoon the sauce over the cabbage rolls. Cover and bake for 1 hour, or until cooked thoroughly. Serve with sauce spooned over each serving.

Cajun Club Sandwich

This sandwich originally went by the name of Cajun Tofu Club, but then we realized that a number of readers wouldn't even look at this recipe if it had tofu in the title. That would have been a shame, because this is such a fantastic sandwich. If you are so tofu-averse that you aren't willing to try this, you can substitute 3 ounces of no-salt-added turkey breast instead.

- 3 or 4 slices low-fat firm tofu, ¼-inch thick (about 3 ounces)
- Canola cooking spray
- 1 teaspoon No-Salt Cajun Spice Mix (page 215) or commercial no-salt Cajun seasoning
- 3 slices light whole wheat or white bread
- 1 tablespoon fat-free mayonnaise
- Red or green leaf lettuce
- 3 to 4 thin slices of tomato

Lay the tofu slices out on a plate and spray both sides lightly with cooking spray. Sprinkle both sides with Cajun Spice Mix and press into the tofu with the back of a spoon. Heat a medium nonstick skillet over medium-high heat. Away from the heat source, spray with cooking spray and return to the heat. Add the tofu in a single layer. Cook for 3 minutes, then flip and cook for another 3 minutes, or until the tofu is firm to the touch, the edges are somewhat crisp, and the seasonings have browned. Remove from the skillet and set aside.

Toast the bread. Lay 1 slice of bread on a cutting board. Spread a little mayonnaise on the side of the bread that is facing up, then top with lettuce and tomato. Top with another slice of toasted

Yield: 1 serving

**Nutritional Information
Per Serving (1 sandwich):**

Calories: 340
Fat: 5.4 g
  Saturated Fat: 1.1 g
  Monounsaturated Fat: 1.7 g
  Polyunsaturated Fat: 2 g
Cholesterol: 0 mg
Sodium: 416 mg
Carbohydrate: 48 g
Dietary Fiber: 7.4 g
Sugars: 3.9 g
Starches: 1.1 g
Protein: 27.3 g
Diabetic Exchanges:
  3 Starch/Bread, 2 Very Lean Meat, ½ Fat

white bread and place the Cajun tofu slices on top of that. Spread a little mayonnaise on the last slice of bread and place it on top of the tofu, mayonnaise side down, to finish off the sandwich. Cut the sandwich into four quarters, slicing from corner to corner, and serve.

Grilled Veggie Sandwich

This sandwich isn't really grilled in the traditional sense, but it is a flavorful, fat-reduced version of a grilled vegetarian sandwich and it makes a great lunch. If desired, you can try it with a little bit of our Zesty Dipping Sauce (page 211) or Tzatziki Sauce (page 210).

Canola cooking spray
¼ cup thinly sliced yellow onion
1 cup thinly sliced white mushrooms
2 tablespoons sliced roasted red pepper
1 ounce shredded reduced-sodium, reduced-fat
    Cheddar cheese
2 slices light whole wheat or multigrain bread
3 to 4 thin slices of tomato
¼ cup alfalfa sprouts

Yield: 1 serving

Nutritional Information Per Serving (1 sandwich):
Calories: 232
Fat: 4.4 g
  Saturated Fat: 1.7 g
  Monounsaturated Fat: 1 g
  Polyunsaturated Fat: 1 g
Cholesterol: 6 mg
Sodium: 383 mg
Carbohydrate: 35.5 g
Dietary Fiber: 4 g
Sugars: 3.9 g
Starches: 0.3 g
Protein: 14.1 g
Diabetic Exchanges:
  1 Starch/Bread, 4 Vegetable,
  1 Fat

Heat a large nonstick skillet over medium heat. Away from the heat source, spray with cooking spray. Return to the heat, add the onion and mushrooms, and cook until onions are soft and mushrooms are tender, about 7 minutes. Stir in the red pepper and cheese and set aside.

Lightly toast the bread. Spoon the vegetable mixture onto 1 slice of bread and top with a layer of sliced tomato and sprouts. Place the second slice of bread on top and cut the sandwich diagonally. Serve immediately.

Rachael Sandwich

Sliced turkey breast is layered with sauerkraut, Swiss cheese, and dressing on slices of toasted rye bread and served warm. This sandwich is a lighter alternative to a Reuben, which is traditionally made with corned beef. And since we are not grilling it using butter, this sandwich is much easier to make, taking only a few minutes. It's also much lower in fat.

1 tablespoon fat-free Thousand Island dressing
3 ounces no-salt-added, low-sodium, reduced-fat
deli-sliced turkey breast
⅓ cup low-sodium sauerkraut, drained
2 slices rye bread
1 slice reduced-fat, low-salt Swiss cheese

Microwave the sliced turkey and the sauerkraut for 1 minute, or until hot.

Lightly toast the rye bread. Top 1 slice of toasted bread with the hot turkey, followed by the cheese and then the sauerkraut. Spread the dressing on the other slice of toasted bread and place facedown on the sauerkraut. Cut the sandwich in half and serve hot.

Yield: 1 serving

**Nutritional Information
Per Serving (1 sandwich):**

Calories: 274
Fat: 4.3 g
 Saturated Fat: 1.7 g
 Monounsaturated Fat: 1.1 g
 Polyunsaturated Fat: 0.8 g
Cholesterol: 60 mg
Sodium: 848 mg
Carbohydrate: 26.1 g
Dietary Fiber: 6.7 g
Sugars: 0 g
Starches: 0.4 g
Protein: 31.1 g
Diabetic Exchanges:
 2 Starch/Bread, 3 Very Lean
 Meat

Cornmeal-Coated Chicken Sandwich

Boneless chicken breast is lightly coated with cornmeal and baked until crispy on the outside and moist on the inside and is served as a sandwich topped with a zesty sauce. Cornmeal is a flour ground from dried corn kernels.

1 3-ounce boneless, skinless chicken breast fillet, fat trimmed
1 egg white
⅓ cup cornmeal
Canola cooking spray
1 whole wheat Kaiser roll, split
Lettuce leaves
Sliced tomato
Sliced red onion
1 tablespoon Cajun Tartar Sauce (page 208) or Creamy Creole Dip (page 212), optional

Preheat oven to 375 degrees F.

Place the chicken and egg white in a bowl and stir to coat.

Place the cornmeal on a plate. Shake excess egg white off the chicken, then lightly coat with cornmeal. Spray both sides of the coated chicken with cooking spray; place on a baking sheet and bake for 10 to 15 minutes, or until cooked through.

Serve the chicken on the Kaiser roll topped with lettuce, tomato, onion, and Cajun Tartar Sauce or Creamy Creole Dip, if desired.

Yield: 1 serving

Nutritional Information Per Serving (1 sandwich):

Calories: 304
Fat: 4.5 g
  Saturated Fat: 0.9 g
  Monounsaturated Fat: 1.1 g
  Polyunsaturated Fat: 1.8 g
Cholesterol: 48 mg
Sodium: 236 mg
Carbohydrate: 39.4 g
Dietary Fiber: 5.3 g
Sugars: 1.1 g
Starch: 1.1 g
Protein: 27.6 g
Diabetic Exchanges:
  2½ Starch/Bread, 3 Very Lean Meat

Chicken Cordon Bleu Sandwich

This simple-to-prepare sandwich version of the renowned classic makes a great lunch item. Traditional Chicken Cordon Bleu is a French dish that tops a thin piece of chicken with ham or prosciutto, gruyère cheese, and herbs before lightly breading and sautéing in butter.

1 egg white
1 3-ounce boneless, skinless chicken breast fillet, fat trimmed
⅓ cup unseasoned bread crumbs
Canola cooking spray
1 thin slice 97% fat-free, low-salt deli-sliced ham
1 thin slice low-fat, low-salt Swiss cheese
1 whole wheat Kaiser roll, split
Lettuce leaves, optional
Sliced tomato, optional
Sliced red onion, optional
1 tablespoon Simple Sour Cream and Dijon Sauce (page 212) or Dijon mustard, optional

Preheat oven to 375 degrees F.

Place the chicken and egg white in a bowl and stir to coat.

Place the bread crumbs on a plate. Shake excess egg white off the chicken, then lightly coat with bread crumbs. Spray both sides of the coated chicken with cooking spray. Place on a baking sheet and bake for 10 to 15 minutes, or until cooked through. Top with the ham and cheese and bake until the cheese melts.

Serve on the Kaiser roll topped with lettuce, tomato, onion, and Simple Sour Cream and Dijon Sauce or Dijon mustard, if desired.

Yield: 1 serving

**Nutritional Information
Per Serving (1 sandwich):**

Calories: 376
Fat: 8.1 g
  Saturated Fat: 2.7 g
  Monounsaturated Fat: 2.4 g
  Polyunsaturated Fat: 2 g
Cholesterol: 64 mg
Sodium: 415 mg
Carbohydrate: 39.6 g
Dietary Fiber: 5 g
Sugars: 0.7 g
Starch: 1.1 g
Protein: 36.9 g
Diabetic Exchanges:
  2 Starch/Bread, 4 Very Lean
  Meat, 1 Fat

Meatball Heroes

Hoagies, heroes, subs, grinders—whatever you call them in your neck of the woods, one thing everyone will call these is delicious. The meatballs and sauce can be prepared ahead of time and stored in the freezer for a quick-to-the-table meatball hero. This recipe can easily be adapted for one serving.

8 meatballs using Classic Italian Meatballs in
   Pomodoro Sauce recipe (page 132)
4 6-inch sub rolls, with or without seeds, sliced in
   half lengthwise
Canola or olive oil cooking spray
½ teaspoon dried parsley flakes
⅓ cup shredded part-skim mozzarella cheese
1 tablespoon grated Parmesan or Romano cheese,
   optional

**Yield: 4 hero sandwiches,
1 sandwich per serving**

**Nutritional Information
Per Serving (1 sandwich):**

Calories: 375
Fat: 8.9 g
   Saturated Fat: 3.5 g
   Monounsaturated Fat: 2.5 g
   Polyunsaturated Fat: 0.9 g
Cholesterol: 45 mg
Sodium: 564 mg
Carbohydrate: 46 g
Dietary Fiber: 3.3 g
Sugars: 0.4 g
Starches: 0.2 g
Protein: 27.2 g
Diabetic Exchanges:
   1 Starch/Bread, 2 Vegetable,
   2 Medium-Fat Meat

Prepare the meatballs and sauce. If you are using previously made meatballs, heat them in a saucepan over medium heat with enough sauce to cover. Cook until the meatballs are heated through. You can also reheat them with the sauce in the microwave, if preferred.

Preheat oven to 400 degrees F.

Lightly spray the cut sides of the sub rolls with cooking spray and sprinkle with the parsley. Place the roll bottoms on a baking sheet, cut side up, and bake until crisp around the edges, about 5 minutes.

Slice the meatballs in half and place 4 halves, cut side down, on each roll bottom. Top with ¼ cup sauce and sprinkle with the shredded mozzarella cheese. Return to the oven along with the roll tops, cut side facing up. Bake for 10 minutes, or until the cheese melts and the top roll is crisp. Sprinkle with Parmesan or Romano cheese, if desired, and serve hot.

8

Side Dishes

Asparagus with Garlic-Shallot Vinaigrette

Asparagus with Lemon-Caper Sauce

Sesame Baby Bok Choy

Spicy Chinese Eggplant

Basil Green Beans

Fresh Green Beans and Red Potatoes Dijon

Green Beans Almondine

Szechuan Snow Peas

Brussels Sprouts Dominique

Ginger-Lime Sugar Snap Peas

Orange-Glazed Carrots

Apple-Cinnamon Carrots

Lemon-Garlic Broccoli Rabe

Zucchini Sautéed with Garlic and Pepper

Grilled Vegetables

Pan-Steamed Spinach with Raisins and Walnuts

Lemon-Spinach Orzo

Baby Peas with Fresh Mint

Collards with Black-Eyed Peas

Refried Black Beans

Pizza Tomatoes

Sweet Potato Fries

Baked French Fries

Roasted Herbed Potatoes

Mock Mashed Potatoes

Cauliflower Lyonnaise

Sweet Potatoes à l'Orange

Whipped Butternut Squash

Holiday Squash

Florentine Rice

Seasoned Basmati Rice

Wild Rice Porcini

Lemon Couscous

Whole Wheat Irish Soda Bread

Sometimes it seems as though side dishes don't get the respect they deserve. It's too bad when you stop to think about it, because side dishes are such an integral part of a complete meal. Side dishes are extremely versatile and can include items such as rice and other grains, pasta, potatoes, and vegetables, as well as fruit and legumes. Side dishes also give you the opportunity to use ingredients that are in season, like Zucchini Sautéed with Garlic and Pepper or Ginger-Lime Sugar Snap Peas during the summer and Whipped Butternut Squash or Apple-Cinnamon Carrots during the Fall.

Many of the side dishes we feature are suitable for a wide range of meals, such as Basil Green Beans and Grilled Vegetables, while others are a bit limited as to what they can be paired with, such as Spicy Chinese Eggplant and Szechuan Snow Peas. Some side dishes can be modified into a main dish, such as Sesame Baby Bok Choy, which can be served with steamed rice and a serving of Asian Cabbage Salad.

Not all vegetables are treated the same nutritionally. Vegetables are split into two types of exchanges for diabetes meal planning, Vegetable and Starch. Vegetable exchanges include such foods as carrots, lettuce, asparagus, zucchini, and broccoli. Starch exchanges include potatoes, peas, winter squash, yams, and corn. Rice, pasta, and grains are also considered a starch, with ½ cup serving being equal to 1 Starch exchange.

Salads can also serve as side dishes. Several salads worthy of side dish status, or at least an honorable mention, are featured in chapter 6. Think about including items such as Creamy Coleslaw, Corn and Black Bean Salad, or Carrot Salad alongside your main dish.

Short on time and long on vegetables? Steam them! Steamed vegetables are among the simplest side dishes you can include with a meal. When in doubt, grab some fresh veggies and steam them until just tender. Add a pinch of dried herbs as seasoning and you're good to go.

Asparagus with Garlic-Shallot Vinaigrette

Asparagus is a good source of folic acid and a significant source of potassium, thiamin, and vitamins A, B_6, and C. When selecting fresh asparagus, look for firm spears with closed, compact tips and a uniform thickness so that they will cook evenly.

Canola cooking spray
½ teaspoon olive oil
1 small shallot, sliced (about 1 tablespoon)
2 cloves garlic, sliced
2 tablespoons fresh-squeezed lemon juice
1 tablespoon balsamic vinegar
Pinch freshly ground black pepper
Pinch dried rosemary, crumbled
1 pound asparagus, tough ends trimmed and stems peeled

Heat a small nonstick skillet over medium heat. Away from the heat source, spray with cooking spray and add oil. Return to the heat, add the shallot, and cook until it softens, about 3 minutes. Add the garlic and sauté for 1 minute. Remove to a small bowl. Add the lemon juice, balsamic vinegar, black pepper, and rosemary; mix well.

Place a metal steamer basket in a large skillet and bring ½ inch of water to a boil. Add the asparagus and steam, covered, until fork-tender, about 4 minutes. Remove the steamed asparagus and arrange on a serving platter. Spoon the garlic-shallot vinaigrette over the cooked asparagus and serve.

Yield: 4 servings

Nutritional Information Per Serving (¼ of recipe):

Calories: 36
Fat: 0.8 g
  Saturated Fat: 0.1 g
  Monounsaturated Fat: 0.4 g
  Polyunsaturated Fat: 0.1 g
Cholesterol: 0 g
Sodium: 4 mg
Carbohydrate: 6.7 g
Dietary Fiber: 2 g
Sugars: 1.1 g
Starches: 0.5 g
Protein: 2.3 g
Diabetic Exchanges:
  1 Vegetable

Asparagus with Lemon-Caper Sauce

*A chilled version of this dish makes a tasty spring salad.
Just replace the broth with 1 tablespoon extra-virgin
olive oil and whisk with the other ingredients in a small
bowl (instead of cooking). Cool the steamed asparagus
under cool water, drain, toss with the dressing, and chill
in the refrigerator for at least an hour, covered.*

Yield: 2 servings

½ pound fresh asparagus, trimmed, cut into thirds
    diagonally
¼ cup Homemade Chicken Broth (page 66) or
    reduced-sodium, low-fat chicken broth
2 tablespoons lemon juice
1 tablespoon capers, rinsed and chopped
1 tablespoon minced fresh parsley
Lemon slices

**Nutritional Information
Per Serving (½ of recipe):**

Calories: 40
Fat: 0.4 g
  Saturated Fat: 0.1 g
  Monounsaturated Fat: 0 g
  Polyunsaturated Fat: 0.1 g
Cholesterol: 0 g
Sodium: 137 mg
Carbohydrate: 8.2 g
Dietary Fiber: 3.4 g
Sugars: 0.4 g
Starches: 0.5 g
Protein: 3.7 g
Diabetic Exchanges:
  2 Vegetable

Steam the asparagus until fork-tender, about 4
minutes.

In a large skillet, heat the broth and lemon juice
over medium-high heat until it begins to boil. Stir
in the capers and cook for 30 seconds, stirring. Add
the steamed asparagus and parsley and toss to
coat.

Remove the asparagus to a serving plate; top
with the remaining sauce and garnish with a few
thin slices of lemon.

Sesame Baby Bok Choy

This is a wonderful accompaniment for any Asian dish or meal. Bok choy, a cabbage widely used in Asian cuisine, is high in calcium and vitamins A and C. When shopping, select fresh bok choy that has firm white stalks and crisp green leaves. This recipe can be used as a main dish for two people by serving 4 bok choy halves over ½ cup of cooked rice per person.

Yield: 4 servings, 2 bok choy halves per serving

Nutritional Information Per Serving (2 bok choy halves):

Calories: 63
Fat: 3.4 g
  Saturated Fat: 0.4 g
  Monounsaturated Fat: 1.2 g
  Polyunsaturated Fat: 1.5 g
Cholesterol: 0 g
Sodium: 220 mg
Carbohydrate: 6.8 g
Dietary Fiber: 2.4 g
Sugars: 1.2 g
Starches: 0 g
Protein: 3.8 g
Diabetic Exchanges:
  1 Vegetable, 1 Fat

¼ cup Homemade Chicken Broth (page 66) or reduced-sodium, low-fat chicken broth
1 tablespoon reduced-sodium teriyaki sauce
½ teaspoon sesame oil
Canola cooking spray
2 teaspoons canola oil
4 baby bok choy, each halved lengthwise, rinsed and patted dry
2 cloves garlic, peeled and minced
2 teaspoons minced fresh ginger
2 scallions, trimmed, and thinly sliced
2 teaspoons toasted sesame seeds

In a small bowl, combine the chicken broth, teriyaki sauce, and sesame oil; set aside.

Over medium-high heat, heat a wok or nonstick skillet for 2 minutes. Away from the heat source, spray the pan with cooking spray. Return tot he heat and add the canola oil. Using tongs, carefully place the bok choy in the pan, cut sides facing up, and brown for 2 minutes. Flip each piece of bok choy over and brown for 1 minute. Remove to a dish and set aside.

Reduce heat to medium and add the garlic and ginger. Cook for about 30 seconds, stirring constantly. Add the chicken broth mixture and simmer for 10 to 15 seconds.

Return the bok choy to the wok, cut sides facing down, and cook for 2 minutes. Add half the sliced scallions and half the sesame seeds. Flip the bok choy over and cook for another minute, or until they are fork tender and the liquid has reduced and thickened slightly.

Remove the bok choy to a serving dish and sprinkle with the remaining sesame seeds and sliced scallions. Serve immediately.

Spicy Chinese Eggplant

A common dish at Chinese buffets, this healthier version can easily be made at home and is just as savory and delicious. Hoisin sauce is a sweet and somewhat spicy sauce made with garlic and chili peppers that is widely used in Chinese cooking and as a condiment. It can usually be found in the ethnic section of major supermarkets. We use crushed red pepper flakes for added heat, but you can omit them for a milder version.

4 Chinese or baby eggplants
2 tablespoons reduced-sodium soy sauce
2 tablespoons Hoisin sauce
½ teaspoon crushed red pepper flakes
½ cup dry sherry
1½ cups water
1 tablespoon canola oil
2 tablespoons minced garlic
2 tablespoons minced fresh ginger
1 teaspoon sesame seeds

Slice the ends off the unpeeled eggplant. Cut each eggplant in half lengthwise, and cut each eggplant half into ¾-inch slices.

Combine the soy sauce, Hoisin sauce, pepper flakes, sherry, and water.

Heat the canola oil in a wok or large skillet. Add the eggplant and stir-fry over high heat for 5 minutes. Add the garlic and ginger and stir-fry for another minute. Add the soy sauce mixture and toss well. Reduce heat to low and simmer for 15 minutes. Remove to a serving platter and sprinkle with the sesame seeds. Serve immediately.

Yield: 6 servings

**Nutritional Information
Per Serving (⅙ of recipe):**

Calories: 110
Fat: 2.8 g
  Saturated Fat: 0.3 g
  Monounsaturated Fat: 1 g
  Polyunsaturated Fat: 1.2 g
Cholesterol: 0 g
Sodium: 291 mg
Carbohydrate: 15.4 g
Dietary Fiber: 5 g
Sugars: 2.2 g
Starches: 0.2 g
Protein: 2.6 g
Diabetic Exchanges:
  3 Vegetable, ½ Fat

Basil Green Beans

Green beans are also commonly called string beans and snap beans. Select fresh beans that are firm and brightly colored and cook only until fork-tender. Green beans are a good source of vitamin A and potassium.

1 pound fresh green beans, ends trimmed, cut into thirds
1 teaspoon olive oil
1 shallot, minced
2 tablespoons chopped fresh basil
Freshly ground black pepper, to taste

Steam the green beans until fork-tender, about 5 minutes.

Meanwhile, in a large skillet, heat the oil over medium-low heat. Add the shallot and sauté until tender, about 4 minutes. Add the basil and sauté for 30 seconds, stirring.

Add the steamed beans to the skillet and toss to coat. Season lightly with freshly ground black pepper and serve hot.

Yield: 4 servings

Nutritional Information Per Serving (½ cup):

Calories: 31
Fat: 1.2 g
 Saturated Fat: 0.2 g
 Monounsaturated Fat: 0.8 g
 Polyunsaturated Fat: 0.1 g
Cholesterol: 0 g
Sodium: 4 mg
Carbohydrate: 4.8 g
Dietary Fiber: 2.1 g
Sugars: 0.2 g
Starches: 0.6 g
Protein: 1.2 g
Diabetic Exchanges:
 1 Vegetable

Fresh Green Beans and Red Potatoes Dijon

This European-style side dish is delicious served warm or cold, and is perfect for a spring picnic.

½ pound small red potatoes, peeled
½ pound fresh green beans, ends trimmed, cut into 1-inch pieces (about 2 cups)
1 tablespoon chopped scallions
1½ tablespoons cider vinegar
2 teaspoons olive oil
1 tablespoon Dijon mustard

Yield: 4 servings

Nutritional Information Per Serving (¼ of recipe):

Calories: 59
Fat: 2.5 g
 Saturated Fat: 0.3 g
 Monounsaturated Fat: 1.7 g
 Polyunsaturated Fat: 0.2 g
Cholesterol: 0 g
Sodium: 97 mg
Carbohydrate: 8.4 g
Dietary Fiber: 3.7 g
Sugars: 0.9 g
Starches: 1.4 g
Protein: 2.5 g
Diabetic Exchanges:
 ½ Starch/Bread

Bring a large pot of water to a boil. Add the potatoes and cook for 5 minutes. Add the green beans and continue to cook until the potatoes and green beans are fork-tender, about 5 more minutes. Drain and transfer to a large bowl and toss with the scallions.

In a small bowl, whisk together the vinegar, olive oil, and mustard. Pour over the beans and potatoes and toss until well coated.

Serve warm as a side dish, or cover and refrigerate until chilled and serve as a summer salad.

Green Beans Almondine

When the name of a dish includes the term amandine *or* almondine, *the dish contains almonds. Almonds are mild in flavor and are a good source of vitamin E, magnesium, and riboflavin. This dish is easy to make and goes very well alongside a mildly flavored fish or poultry dish.*

½ pound green beans, ends trimmed diagonally, cut in half diagonally
Canola cooking spray
1 teaspoon light margarine
2 tablespoons sliced almonds
Salt substitute
Freshly ground black pepper

Steam green beans until fork-tender. Heat a large nonstick skillet over medium heat. Away from the heat source, spray with cooking spray. Return to the heat source and melt the margarine. Add the almonds and cook for 2 minutes or until golden, stirring often.

Add the green beans to the skillet and toss with the almonds. Season with salt substitute and black pepper, to taste. Serve hot.

Yield: 2 servings, can be doubled

Nutritional Information Per Serving (½ of recipe):

Calories: 79
Fat: 4.4 g
  Saturated Fat: 0.5 g
  Monounsaturated Fat: 2.4 g
  Polyunsaturated Fat: 1.1 g
Cholesterol: 0 g
Sodium: 20 mg
Carbohydrate: 9.1 g
Dietary Fiber: 4.4 g
Sugars: 0 g
Starches: 0 g
Protein: 3.3 g
Diabetic Exchanges:
  2 Vegetable, 1 Fat

Szechuan Snow Peas

Szechuan, or Sichuan, cuisine originates from the Sichuan province of western China. It has a reputation for being very spicy. A popular example served in restaurants is Kung Pao Chicken. Szechuan cuisine features many mildly flavored dishes, but this version of Szechuan Snow Peas is not one of them. This is a spicy three-ingredient recipe that you can make in under 5 minutes. Try it alongside some rice and grilled seafood for a nice meal. Ground chili paste can be found in most major supermarkets in the Asian or ethnic foods area. You can substitute crushed red pepper flakes instead, if necessary.

½ cup Homemade Chicken Broth (page 66) or
 Homemade Vegetable Broth (page 68)
1 teaspoon prepared ground chili paste
1 pound fresh snow peas, ends trimmed

Bring the broth and chili paste to a boil in a large skillet over medium-high heat. Add the snow peas and cook, covered, until the snow peas wilt and become tender, about 3 minutes. Toss to coat and serve hot.

Yield: 4 servings, about ½ cup per serving

Nutritional Information Per Serving (½ cup):

Calories: 29
Fat: 0.2 g
 Saturated Fat: 0.5 g
 Monounsaturated Fat: 0 g
 Polyunsaturated Fat: 0.1 g
Cholesterol: 0 mg
Sodium: 7 mg
Carbohydrate: 5.2 g
Dietary Fiber: 1.8 g
Sugars: 0 g
Starches: 0 g
Protein: 1.9 g
Diabetic Exchanges:
 1 Vegetable

Brussels Sprouts Dominique

Brussels sprouts, named after the capital of Belgium, resemble small heads of cabbage, have a similar, but milder, taste, and are high in vitamin C. Select brussels sprouts that are firm and bright green.

1 pound brussels sprouts, trimmed
Canola cooking spray
½ teaspoon canola oil
1 shallot, minced
½ cup sliced scallions
2 tablespoons dry vermouth or dry white wine
2 tablespoons water
½ cup red seedless grapes, halved

Yield: 4 servings, about ½ cup per serving

Nutritional Information Per Serving (½ cup):

Calories: 64
Fat: 0.9 g
 Saturated Fat: 0.9 g
 Monounsaturated Fat: 0.3 g
 Polyunsaturated Fat: 0.4 g
Cholesterol: 0 mg
Sodium: 25 mg
Carbohydrate: 11.8 g
Dietary Fiber: 3.9 g
Sugars: 2.1 g
Starches: 0.3 g
Protein: 3.4 g
Diabetic Exchanges:
 1 Vegetable, ½ Fruit

Bring a pot of water to a boil over high heat. Add the brussels sprouts and cook until tender, about 12 minutes. Drain and set aside.

Heat a large nonstick skillet over medium heat. Away from the heat source, spray with cooking spray and add the oil. Return to the heat and sauté the shallot for 2 minutes. Stir in the scallions, wine, water, and grapes and cook for 1 minute, stirring. Add the cooked brussels sprouts and toss to coat.

Ginger-Lime Sugar Snap Peas

This tasty side dish pairs well with grilled seafood or poultry and can easily be doubled. Sugar snap peas are a good source of potassium, calcium, vitamin A, vitamin C, and folate.

Yield: 2 servings, about ½ cup per serving

1 cup fresh sugar snap peas, ends trimmed
Canola cooking spray
½ teaspoon canola oil
1 teaspoon minced garlic
1 tablespoon grated fresh ginger
2 teaspoons lime juice

Steam the sugar snap peas until fork-tender.

Meanwhile, heat a large nonstick skillet over medium-low heat. Away from the heat source, spray with cooking spray and add the oil. Return to the heat, add the garlic and ginger, and sauté for 5 minutes. Stir in the lime juice and swirl around. Add the steamed sugar snap peas and toss to coat.

Nutritional Information Per Serving (½ cup):

Calories: 32
Fat: 1.2 g
  Saturated Fat: 0.1 g
  Monounsaturated Fat: 0.5 g
  Polyunsaturated Fat: 0.5 g
Cholesterol: 0 mg
Sodium: 4 mg
Carbohydrate: 4.7 g
Dietary Fiber: 1.1 g
Sugars: 1.5 g
Starches: 0.2 g
Protein: 1.2 g
Diabetic Exchanges:
  1 Vegetable

Orange-Glazed Carrots

Glazed carrots are especially popular around the holidays. This version is low in fat and sodium and can easily be doubled.

2 cups baby-cut carrots
¼ cup water
2 tablespoons no-pulp orange juice concentrate
1 teaspoon sugar-free pancake syrup

Steam carrots until fork-tender; set aside.

In a large nonstick skillet, heat the water and orange juice concentrate over medium-high heat until it begins to bubble. Reduce heat and add the carrots; heat for 2 minutes, stirring often. Drizzle with pancake syrup and toss well. Serve hot.

Yield: 4 servings, about ½ cup per serving

Nutritional Information Per Serving (½ cup):

Calories: 41
Fat: 0.1 g
  Saturated Fat: 0 g
  Monounsaturated Fat: 0 g
  Polyunsaturated Fat: 0 g
Cholesterol: 0 g
Sodium: 23 mg
Carbohydrate: 9.7 g
Dietary Fiber: 1.9 g
Sugars: 3.4 g
Starches: 0 g
Protein: 0.8 g
Diabetic Exchanges:
  2 Vegetable

Apple-Cinnamon Carrots

This sweet and flavorful dish is perfectly suited for autumn. Try adding some golden raisins and dried cranberries for a festive variation.

2 cups sliced carrots, ¼-inch thick (about 4 medium carrots)
¼ cup water
¼ cup diced peeled Granny Smith apple
¼ teaspoon ground cinnamon
1 teaspoon apple juice concentrate

Steam carrots until fork-tender; set aside.

In a large nonstick skillet, heat the water over medium-high heat until it begins to boil. Add the apple and cinnamon; reduce heat to medium and cook for 30 seconds, stirring. Add the carrots and apple juice concentrate; cook for 1 minute, stirring and tossing until well combined. Serve hot.

Yield: 4 servings, about ½ cup per serving

Nutritional Information Per Serving (½ cup):

Calories: 34
Fat: 0.1 g
  Saturated Fat: 0 g
  Monounsaturated Fat: 0 g
  Polyunsaturated Fat: 0 g
Cholesterol: 0 g
Sodium: 22 mg
Carbohydrate: 8.2 g
Dietary Fiber: 2 g
Sugars: 0.9 g
Starches: 0 g
Protein: 0.7 g
Diabetic Exchanges:
  1 Vegetable

Lemon-Garlic Broccoli Rabe

*Broccoli rabe has a somewhat bitter taste, which mel-
lows a little after cooking, and is a good source of vitamins A, C, and K, as well as beta-carotene. It is popular
in both Chinese and Italian cuisine and is also commonly called raab, rapa, rapine, rappi, or rapini.*

1½ pounds broccoli rabe, preferably thin stemmed,
     washed
¼ cup water
1 teaspoon olive oil
1 teaspoon unsalted butter
1 teaspoon minced garlic
2 tablespoons fresh lemon juice
Freshly ground black pepper, to taste
1 tablespoon minced fresh parsley leaves
1 teaspoon freshly grated lemon zest

Yield: 4 servings

**Nutritional Information
Per Serving (¼ of recipe):**

Calories: 31
Fat: 2.4 g
  Saturated Fat: 0.8 g
  Monounsaturated Fat: 1.1 g
  Polyunsaturated Fat: 0.3 g
Cholesterol: 3 g
Sodium: 16 mg
Carbohydrate: 2.6 g
Dietary Fiber: 1.3 g
Sugars: 0.4 g
Starches: 0.3 g
Protein: 0.6 g
Diabetic Exchanges:
  1 Vegetable, ½ Fat

Remove any discolored leaves from the broccoli
rabe and slice off stem ends.

Heat a large nonstick skillet over medium-high
heat. Add the water and the broccoli rabe and
steam, covered, until the stems are fork-tender.

Meanwhile, heat the oil and butter in a small
nonstick skillet over medium-low heat until the
butter melts. Add the garlic and cook for 2 minutes, stirring occasionally, until the garlic softens.
Stir in the lemon juice, heat for 30 seconds, and set
aside.

When the broccoli rabe is fork-tender, drain and
transfer to a large bowl. Season lightly with freshly
ground black pepper and add the parsley. Pour the
lemon-garlic sauce over the broccoli rabe and toss.
Place the broccoli rabe on a serving dish and spoon
the sauce over it. Sprinkle with grated lemon zest
and serve immediately.

Zucchini Sautéed with Garlic and Pepper

Zucchini has a high water content and can release a substantial amount of liquid while cooking. To prevent the zucchini from becoming soggy, make sure you sauté it until it just becomes tender. You can omit the red pepper flakes called for in this recipe if you would prefer a milder version.

2 teaspoons olive oil
1 pound zucchini, sliced into ¼-inch-thick slices
1 to 2 cloves garlic, minced
¼ teaspoon crushed red pepper flakes
1 tablespoon balsamic vinegar

In a large nonstick skillet, heat the oil over medium-high heat. Add the zucchini slices and sauté for 3 to 4 minutes, or until the zucchini is almost fork-tender. Add the garlic and continue to sauté for 1 minute. Add the red pepper flakes and balsamic vinegar and toss well. Serve immediately.

Yield: 4 servings

**Nutritional Information
Per Serving (¼ of recipe):**

Calories: 37
Fat: 2.4 g
  Saturated Fat: 0.3 g
  Monounsaturated Fat: 1.7 g
  Polyunsaturated Fat: 0.3 g
Cholesterol: 0 g
Sodium: 3 mg
Carbohydrate: 3.9 g
Dietary Fiber: 1.1 g
Sugars: 0.9 g
Starches: 0.2 g
Protein: 1.1 g
Diabetic Exchanges:
  1 Vegetable, ½ Fat

Grilled Vegetables

These grilled vegetables are great right off the grill, but you can also toss them with some balsamic vinegar and olive oil after they are cooked. Make a sandwich using grilled Italian bread and top it with Rocco's Pomodoro Sauce (page 207), Tzatziki Sauce (page 210), Raspberry Vinaigrette (page 216), or House Italian Dressing (page 216).

1 large green zucchini, sliced diagonally into ½-inch rounds
1 large yellow squash, sliced diagonally into ½-inch rounds
1 large red bell pepper, cut into 1-inch strips
1 large eggplant, sliced into ½-inch-thick rounds
Canola oil
Canola or olive oil cooking spray
1 teaspoon no-salt Italian seasoning

Yield: 4 servings

**Nutritional Information
Per Serving (¼ of recipe):**

Calories: 60
Fat: 0.5 g
  Saturated Fat: 0.1 g
  Monounsaturated Fat: 0 g
  Polyunsaturated Fat: 0.2 g
Cholesterol: 0 g
Sodium: 8 mg
Carbohydrate: 13.8 g
Dietary Fiber: 5.3 g
Sugars: 0 g
Starches: 0 g
Protein: 2.9 g
Diabetic Exchanges:
  2 Vegetable

Heat a grill until medium-hot (if you use a grill pan, you will have to cook in batches). Lightly oil the grill rack with canola oil using a paper towel. Spray all the vegetables with cooking spray and sprinkle with Italian seasoning. Grill the vegetables until tender, flipping every few minutes for even cooking.

Pan-Steamed Spinach with Raisins and Walnuts

This dish provides a wonderful combination of sweetness from the raisins and savory texture from the walnuts. It is terrific with steamed or baked fish as well as with grilled Mediterranean dishes. Spinach is a rich source of vitamins A and K, folate, and carotenoids such as beta-carotene and lutein. Walnuts contain omega-3 fatty acids, which may help fight heart disease.

Yield: 2 servings

**Nutritional Information
Per Serving (½ of recipe):**

Calories: 114
Fat: 4.9 g
 Saturated Fat: 0.5 g
 Monounsaturated Fat: 2.2 g
 Polyunsaturated Fat: 1.8 g
Cholesterol: 0 g
Sodium: 85 mg
Carbohydrate: 16.4 g
Dietary Fiber: 3.6 g
Sugars: 1.7 g
Starches: 0.3 g
Protein: 4.3 g
Diabetic Exchanges:
 3 Vegetable, 1 Fat

Canola cooking spray
1 teaspoon olive oil
3 tablespoons golden raisins
2 tablespoons coarsely chopped walnuts
1 teaspoon minced garlic
1 tablespoon water
1 10-ounce package fresh spinach, stemmed and
 rinsed
Pinch salt or salt substitute
Freshly ground black pepper, to taste

Heat a nonstick skillet over medium-high heat. Away from the heat source, spray with cooking spray and add the olive oil. Return to the heat, add the raisins and walnuts and cook for 20 seconds, stirring. Add the garlic, water, and spinach; cover and cook for 2 minutes, or until the spinach wilts. Season to taste with salt substitute and ground black pepper and serve.

Lemon-Spinach Orzo

One pound of stemmed fresh spinach can be used for this dish instead of frozen. Just sauté the fresh spinach with the garlic until it wilts, then add the orzo.

⅓ cup orzo, uncooked
Canola cooking spray
½ teaspoon olive oil
1 tablespoon minced garlic
½ teaspoon no-salt Italian seasoning
2 tablespoons lemon juice
1 10-ounce package frozen whole spinach, thawed
Lemon wedges
Pinch salt substitute
Freshly ground black pepper to taste
Grated Romano cheese, optional

Cook orzo according to package directions until al dente, without any added salt or oil. Drain and set aside.

Heat a large nonstick skillet over medium heat. Away from the heat source, coat pan with cooking spray and add the olive oil. Return to the heat, add the garlic and Italian seasoning, and sauté for 30 seconds. Add the lemon juice and swirl around with the garlic. Add the spinach and toss with the garlic. Cook, stirring, for 1 minute, or until the spinach is warm.

Add the cooked orzo to the spinach and stir until well combined. Remove to a serving platter and squeeze the juice from 2 lemon wedges over it. Lightly season with salt substitute and black pepper and sprinkle with Romano cheese, if desired. Garnish with additional lemon wedges.

Yield: 6 servings

**Nutritional Information
Per Serving (⅙ of recipe):**

Calories: 53
Fat: 0.7 g
  Saturated Fat: 0.1 g
  Monounsaturated Fat: 0.3 g
  Polyunsaturated Fat: 0.2 g
Cholesterol: 0 g
Sodium: 37 mg
Carbohydrate: 9.7 g
Dietary Fiber: 1.9 g
Sugars: 0.9 g
Starches: 6.4 g
Protein: 2.7 g
Diabetic Exchanges:
  ½ Starch/Bread, 1 Vegetable

Baby Peas with Fresh Mint

Sweet baby peas team up with lemon zest and fresh mint for a flavorful, easy-to-prepare side dish that pairs well with fish and poultry. Frozen peas keep their deep green color, fresh flavor, and valuable nutrients better than canned peas, plus they do not contain the added sodium. They are also a great low-fat source of protein and dietary fiber and a good source of vitamin C and folate.

Yield: 4 servings

**Nutritional Information
Per Serving (¼ of recipe):**

Calories: 77
Fat: 2.2 g
  Saturated Fat: 0.3 g
  Monounsaturated Fat: 0.7 g
  Polyunsaturated Fat: 0.8 g
Cholesterol: 0 g
Sodium: 75 mg
Carbohydrate: 10.4 g
Dietary Fiber: 3.7 g
Sugars: 0.2 g
Starches: 0.8 g
Protein: 3.5 g
Diabetic Exchanges:
  2 Vegetable, ½ Fat

Canola cooking spray
½ teaspoon canola oil
1 shallot, finely chopped
2 tablespoons dry white wine
½ teaspoon grated lemon zest
1 tablespoon light margarine
1 10-ounce package frozen baby peas, thawed and
    drained
Pinch salt substitute
Pinch freshly ground black pepper
2 or 3 fresh mint leaves, finely sliced (about 1½
    teaspoons)

Heat a large nonstick skillet over medium heat. Away from the heat source, spray skillet with cooking spray and add the oil. Return to the heat and sauté shallot for 1 minute. Add the wine and lemon zest and stir for 10 seconds. Add the margarine and peas and season lightly with salt substitute and black pepper. Stir until well combined and cook until the peas are heated through, about 3 minutes. Add the mint and stir for 30 seconds. Serve hot.

Collards with Black-Eyed Peas

Collards, or collard greens, are a dark green leafy vegetable from the cabbage family. They have a slightly bitter flavor that falls somewhere between kale and cabbage. Black-eyed peas are soft beans that provide a good source of calcium, folate, fiber, and vitamin A. Both collards and black-eyed peas have gained popularity thanks to dishes from the southern United States similar to this one, such as collard greens with ham hocks.

Canola cooking spray
½ teaspoon canola oil
½ cup chopped yellow onion
½ cup diced yellow or orange bell pepper
1 pound collards, cleaned, stems removed, and chopped
1 tablespoon minced garlic
⅓ cup Homemade Chicken Broth (page 66) or reduced-sodium, low-fat chicken broth
1½ cups diced tomatoes
1 15.5-ounce can black-eyed peas, rinsed and drained
2 slices reduced-sodium turkey bacon, cooked crisp and chopped
Freshly ground black pepper to taste

Heat a large nonstick skillet over medium heat. Away from the heat source, coat the pan with cooking spray and add the canola oil. Return to the heat and sauté the onion and bell pepper until the onion softens, about 5 minutes. Add the collards and garlic and cook until the collards are wilted, about 1 minute. Stir in the broth, tomatoes, black-eyed peas, and turkey bacon and season with black pepper. Cover and simmer for 7 minutes over medium-low heat. Serve hot.

Yield: 6 servings

Nutritional Information Per Serving (⅙ of recipe):

Calories: 129
Fat: 2 g
  Saturated Fat: 0.4 g
  Monounsaturated Fat: 0.5 g
  Polyunsaturated Fat: 0.7 g
Cholesterol: 3 g
Sodium: 109 mg
Carbohydrate: 23.9 g
Dietary Fiber: 7.5 g
Sugars: 1.6 g
Starches: 0.3 g
Protein: 6.1 g
Diabetic Exchanges:
  1 Starch/Bread, 2 Vegetable

Refried Black Beans

This easy-to-make, flavorful, low-fat dish is sensational with Mexican or southwestern-style dishes, such as our Spicy Southwestern-Style Grilled Chicken (page 41) and Huevos Rancheros (page 99). For some added heat, you can spice it up with diced jalapeño peppers. This dish can also be used as a dip or burrito filling.

Canola cooking spray
½ teaspoon canola oil
¼ cup chopped yellow onion
1 clove garlic, minced
1 15.5-ounce can low-sodium black beans
3 or 4 drops hot pepper sauce, or to taste
½ cup water

Heat a 1-quart saucepan over medium heat. Away from the heat source, spray with cooking spray and add the oil. Return to the heat, add the onion, and sauté until softened, about 5 minutes. Add the garlic and stir for 45 seconds. Stir in the beans, hot sauce, and water and bring to a boil. Reduce heat to low, cover, and simmer for 20 to 25 minutes, stirring vigorously every few minutes to break up the beans. You may need to add water (2 tablespoons at a time) to prevent the beans from drying out or burning. You should be able to stir the bean mixture into a chunky paste. Serve hot.

Yield: 4 servings, can be doubled

Nutritional Information Per Serving (¼ of recipe):
Calories: 108
Fat: 1 g
  Saturated Fat: 0.1 g
  Monounsaturated Fat: 0.3 g
  Polyunsaturated Fat: 0.4 g
Cholesterol: 0 mg
Sodium: 97 mg
Carbohydrate: 18.8 g
Dietary Fiber: 6.7 g
Sugars: 2.5 g
Starches: 9.6 g
Protein: 6.8 g
Diabetic Exchanges:
  1 Starch/Bread

Pizza Tomatoes

These surprisingly easy to make tomatoes are great alongside Mediterranean-style grilled chicken or pork dishes, such as our Italian Roast Pork (page 137). You can also make a pizza sandwich using a few of the tomato slices and Italian bread or serve with Garlic Crostini (page 61) as an appetizer.

Olive oil cooking spray
2 large vine-ripened tomatoes
2 tablespoons unseasoned bread crumbs
1 teaspoon no-salt Italian seasoning
⅛ teaspoon garlic powder
⅛ teaspoon crushed red pepper flakes, optional
¼ cup shredded part-skim mozzarella cheese

Yield: 2 servings, can be doubled

Nutritional Information Per Serving (½ of recipe):
Calories: 94
Fat: 3.2 g
  Saturated Fat: 1.7 g
  Monounsaturated Fat: 0.9 g
  Polyunsaturated Fat: 0.3 g
Cholesterol: 8 mg
Sodium: 146 mg
Carbohydrate: 11.4 g
Dietary Fiber: 1.5 g
Sugars: 0 g
Starches: 0 g
Protein: 5.8 g
Diabetic Exchanges:
  1 Starch/Bread, 1 Vegetable, ½ Fat

Preheat broiler. Line a baking sheet with aluminum foil and spray lightly with cooking spray.

Slice the ends off the tomatoes and cut each tomato into two thick slices.

In a small bowl, combine the bread crumbs, Italian seasoning, garlic powder, and red pepper flakes, if desired. Press the larger side of each slice of tomato into the bread crumb mixture and lay on the baking sheet, crumb side up. Arrange the slices with at least 1 inch between them. Lightly spray the tops of the tomatoes with cooking spray.

Broil the tomatoes at least 8 inches away from the heat source until the bread crumbs brown slightly, about 4 minutes. Remove from the oven and top each tomato with shredded cheese. Broil until the cheese melts and browns slightly, about 2 minutes, and serve hot.

Sweet Potato Fries

This sweet treat is especially good when served alongside grilled or roast chicken or turkey. When eaten with the skin still on, sweet potatoes are a great source of fiber. They also provide good amounts of vitamins C and B_6, as well as beta-carotene.

Yield: 4 servings, can be doubled

Canola cooking spray
3 or 4 sweet potatoes (about 1 pound), unpeeled and scrubbed
Salt substitute, to taste
Freshly ground black pepper, to taste

Nutritional Information Per Serving (¼ of recipe):

Calories: 88
Fat: 0.1 g
  Saturated Fat: 0 g
  Monounsaturated Fat: 0 g
  Polyunsaturated Fat: 0.1 g
Cholesterol: 0 g
Sodium: 9 mg
Carbohydrate: 20.8 g
Dietary Fiber: 2.6 g
Sugars: 9.7 g
Starches: 8.5 g
Protein: 1.5 g
Diabetic Exchanges:
  1½ Starch/Bread

Preheat oven to 425 degrees F. Line a baking sheet with aluminum foil and spray with cooking spray.

Cut the sweet potatoes, with the skin still on, into long ½-inch-thick strips; discard any tiny pieces that are left over.

Place the sweet potato fries in a large mixing bowl. Spray with cooking spray, toss well, then spray again so that all the fries are lightly coated.

Arrange the fries on the baking sheet with space between them. Bake for 10 minutes. Remove from the oven and flip the fries over with a spatula. Return to the oven and bake for another 10 minutes, or until crisp. Lightly season with salt substitute and black pepper, to taste.

Baked French Fries

These French fries are simple to make and much healthier than fast-food fries or the kind you might find in the frozen food aisle. You can also spice these up by sprinkling them with No-Salt Cajun Spice Mix (page 215) or Creole Seasoning Mix (page 215) before you put them in the oven.

Yield: 4 servings

Nutritional Information Per Serving (¼ of recipe):
Calories: 130
Fat: 0 g
  Saturated Fat: 0 g
  Monounsaturated Fat: 0 g
  Polyunsaturated Fat: 0.1 g
Cholesterol: 0 g
Sodium: 12 mg
Carbohydrate: 29.3 g
Dietary Fiber: 3.3 g
Sugars: 2.8 g
Starches: 23.3 g
Protein: 3.9 g
Diabetic Exchanges:
  2 Starch/Bread

  4 medium baking potatoes, scrubbed and cut
      lengthwise into ½-inch-wide strips, unpeeled
  Canola cooking spray
  ½ teaspoon salt substitute, optional

Preheat oven to 375 degrees F.

In a large bowl, soak the cut potatoes in cold water for 5 minutes. Drain and pat dry with cloth or paper towels. Towel dry the mixing bowl and return the potatoes to it. Spray the potatoes with cooking spray, tossing every few sprays so all sides are lightly coated.

Spread the potatoes out in a single layer on a large baking sheet. Bake until golden and just crisp, about 30 minutes, turning once with a spatula after about 15 minutes. If you prefer crispier fries, bake them a little longer.

Sprinkle the fries with the salt substitute, if desired, and divide into 4 portions. Serve hot.

Roasted Herbed Potatoes

Roasted Herbed Potatoes can be used as a side dish for breakfast, lunch, or dinner. You can even toss them with a light vinaigrette to serve as a warm or cold salad. Leftovers can be reheated in the microwave until hot.

12 small new potatoes, scrubbed and halved, unpeeled
Olive oil cooking spray
2 cloves garlic, chopped
¼ teaspoon freshly ground black pepper
1 tablespoon finely chopped fresh flat-leaf parsley
2 tablespoons chopped scallions

Preheat oven to 350 degrees F.

In a large mixing bowl, spray the potatoes with olive oil spray. Toss with the garlic and black pepper. Place in a shallow roasting dish and roast until the potatoes are cooked through and become just crisp and golden brown in color, about 30 minutes. Remove to a large mixing bowl and toss well with the parsley and scallions.

Yield: 4 servings

Nutritional Information Per Serving (¼ of recipe):

Calories: 152
Fat: 0.2 g
  Saturated Fat: 0 g
  Monounsaturated Fat: 0 g
  Polyunsaturated Fat: 0.1 g
Cholesterol: 0 g
Sodium: 13 mg
Carbohydrate: 34.7 g
Dietary Fiber: 3.2 g
Sugars: 0.4 g
Starches: 34.3 g
Protein: 4.1 g
Diabetic Exchanges:
  2 Starch/Bread

Mock Mashed Potatoes

This delicious bit of culinary trickery is especially handy during the holidays. It may sound crazy, but many people actually believe they are eating potatoes. By using cauliflower, you can enjoy a lower-carbohydrate alternative to potatoes that goes just as well with roast chicken, turkey, and meat. Serve with our Homemade Gravy (page 209) or Savory Mushroom Gravy (page 208), if desired.

1 medium head cauliflower, chopped
⅓ cup light sour cream
½ teaspoon salt substitute, or to taste
⅛ teaspoon white pepper, or to taste

Yield: 4 servings

Nutritional Information Per Serving (¼ of recipe):

Calories: 47
Fat: 2.3 g
  Saturated Fat: 1.4 g
  Monounsaturated Fat: 0.6 g
  Polyunsaturated Fat: 0.2 g
Cholesterol: 7 g
Sodium: 37 mg
Carbohydrate: 5.4 g
Dietary Fiber: 1.9 g
Sugars: 1.8 g
Starches: 0.2 g
Protein: 2.2 g
Diabetic Exchanges:
  1 Vegetable, ½ Fat

Steam or boil the cauliflower in a large pot until very soft and drain well; let sit until cool enough to handle.

Run the cauliflower through a food mill or ricer or process using the shredder attachment on a food processor. Remove to a large bowl and stir in the remaining ingredients. Serve hot.

Cauliflower Lyonnaise

This recipe was inspired by Potatoes Lyonnaise, a French classic that combines potatoes, onion, butter, and fresh herbs. It serves well as a side dish for brunch or dinner.

Yield: 4 servings

Nutritional Information Per Serving (¼ of recipe):

Calories: 58
Fat: 3 g
  Saturated Fat: 1.2 g
  Monounsaturated Fat: 1.3 g
  Polyunsaturated Fat: 0.3 g
Cholesterol: 5 g
Sodium: 20 mg
Carbohydrate: 6.7 g
Dietary Fiber: 2 g
Sugars: 0.2 g
Starches: 0 g
Protein: 1.9 g
Diabetic Exchanges:
  1 Vegetable, 1 Fat

1 medium head cauliflower, chopped
Canola or olive oil cooking spray
1 teaspoon olive oil
1 cup chopped yellow onion
1 clove garlic, minced
1 tablespoon chopped fresh parsley, or 1 teaspoon dried parsley flakes
¼ cup light sour cream
½ teaspoon salt substitute, or to taste
⅛ teaspoon ground white pepper, or to taste

Steam or boil cauliflower in a large pot until very soft and drain well.

Meanwhile, heat a large saucepan over medium heat. Away from the heat source, spray with cooking spray and add the oil. Return to the heat and sauté the onion until soft, 5 to 7 minutes. Add the garlic and parsley and sauté for 1 minute.

Stir in the sour cream, then add the cauliflower, salt substitute, and white pepper. Stir until heated through and well combined. Serve immediately.

Sweet Potatoes à l'Orange

The natural sweetness of the potatoes teams up with orange juice, zest, and pancake syrup for an easy-to-prepare dish well suited for baked ham and holiday menus. It is also a great low-fat, cholesterol-free source of fiber and vitamin C.

Canola cooking spray
1½ pounds sweet potatoes, peeled and sliced
    ½-inch thick
½ cup orange juice
¼ teaspoon cinnamon
2 tablespoons minced orange zest
2 tablespoons sugar-free pancake syrup

Preheat oven to 375 degrees F. Coat a 13-by-9-by-2-inch casserole or baking dish with cooking spray.

Arrange sweet potato slices in layers in the casserole. Pour the orange juice over the potatoes. Sprinkle with the cinnamon and orange zest and drizzle with the pancake syrup. Cover casserole and bake for 30 minutes, or until the sweet potatoes are tender. Serve hot.

Yield: 8 servings

**Nutritional Information
Per Serving (⅛ of recipe):**

Calories: 78
Fat: 0.1 g
  Saturated Fat: 0 g
  Monounsaturated Fat: 0 g
  Polyunsaturated Fat: 0.1 g
Cholesterol: 0 g
Sodium: 10 mg
Carbohydrate: 18.4 g
Dietary Fiber: 2.1 g
Sugars: 9.3 g
Starches: 6.9 g
Protein: 1.3 g
Diabetic Exchanges: 1
  Starch/Bread

Whipped Butternut Squash

Butternut squash is a good low-fat source of fiber, complex carbohydrate, potassium, vitamin C, and beta-carotene. Steaming the squash instead of boiling it can help retain more of the flavor and nutrients, but it will take two to three times longer than boiling.

1 (1 to 1¼ pound) butternut squash, peeled and cut
    into 1-inch cubes
¼ cup light sour cream
¼ cup fat-free skim milk
Pinch salt substitute
Pinch ground black pepper

Steam or boil squash until very tender. Drain and return to the pot, without any heat. Add the sour cream, milk, salt substitute, and black pepper. Using a hand mixer, blend until creamy and smooth. Add more skim milk, 1 tablespoon at a time, if it is too thick for your taste. Serve warm.

Yield: 6 servings

**Nutritional Information
Per Serving (⅙ of recipe):**

Calories: 45
Fat: 0.9 g
  Saturated Fat: 0.5 g
  Monounsaturated Fat: 0.2 g
  Polyunsaturated Fat: 0.1 g
Cholesterol: 3 g
Sodium: 12 mg
Carbohydrate: 9.1 g
Dietary Fiber: 0 g
Sugars: 0.3 g
Starches: 0 g
Protein: 1.2 g
Diabetic Exchanges:
  ½ Starch/Bread

Holiday Squash

This dish combines sweet squash, apple, and walnuts for an autumn side dish that is perfect for the holidays. Baking the acorn squash helps bring out its sweetness as the squash's natural sugars caramelize while it slowly bakes. Acorn squash is a great source of dietary fiber and also provides B vitamins, vitamin C, and potassium, which the body needs for normal cell function.

2 small acorn squash (1½ pounds total), halved
Canola cooking spray
1 large Granny Smith apple, peeled, cored, and chopped
2 tablespoons chopped walnuts
2 tablespoons diced celery
2 tablespoons finely chopped yellow onion
2 teaspoons margarine, melted
2 tablespoons apple cider
Freshly ground pepper, to taste

Preheat oven to 375 degrees F. Lightly spray a baking pan with cooking spray.

Scoop the seeds out of each squash half. Place the squash halves, cut side down, on the baking pan and bake for 25 minutes.

Meanwhile, combine the apple, walnuts, celery, onion, margarine, and cider in a medium bowl.

Remove the squash from the oven and turn each half over. Spoon the apple-walnut mixture into the scooped-out portion of the squash halves and season lightly with black pepper. Cover with aluminum foil and return to the oven; bake for 35 minutes. Serve hot.

Yield: 4 servings, 1 stuffed squash half per serving

Nutritional Information Per Serving (1 stuffed squash half):

Calories: 150
Fat: 4.7 g
  Saturated Fat: 0.6 g
  Monounsaturated Fat: 1.4 g
  Polyunsaturated Fat: 2.3 g
Cholesterol: 0 g
Sodium: 33 mg
Carbohydrate: 28.8 g
Dietary Fiber: 4.3 g
Sugars: 3.4 g
Starches: 0 g
Protein: 2.4 g
Diabetic Exchanges:
  1 Starch/Bread, 2 Vegetable, 1 Fat

Florentine Rice

Rosemary's pinelike flavor complements a number of foods, and fresh rosemary is often paired with roast lamb or poultry. The small amount of dried rosemary used in this dish is just enough to enhance the flavor without overpowering it. Feel free to add chopped fresh tomato as a variation, if desired.

1 teaspoon olive oil
1 teaspoon light margarine
1 medium red bell pepper, seeded and diced
⅓ cup sliced scallions
1 clove garlic, minced
½ pound fresh spinach, cleaned, stemmed, and torn into pieces
¼ teaspoon crushed dried rosemary
¼ teaspoon ground white pepper
2½ cups cooked brown rice
2 tablespoons grated Parmesan cheese

In a large skillet, heat the oil and margarine over medium heat until the margarine melts. Add the red bell pepper and scallions and sauté for 3 minutes. Add the garlic and sauté for 30 seconds. Add the spinach, rosemary, and white pepper and cook until the spinach wilts. Add the brown rice and Parmesan cheese, and stir until rice is heated through and the cheese has melted. Serve hot.

Yield: 6 servings

**Nutritional Information
Per Serving (⅙ of recipe):**

Calories: 124
Fat: 2.6 g
  Saturated Fat: 0.6 g
  Monounsaturated Fat: 1.1 g
  Polyunsaturated Fat: 0.5 g
Cholesterol: 2 g
Sodium: 72 mg
Carbohydrate: 21.6 g
Dietary Fiber: 2.8 g
Sugars: 0.9 g
Starches: 16.6 g
Protein: 4.2 g
Diabetic Exchanges:
  1 Starch/Bread, 1 Vegetable,
  ½ Fat

Seasoned Basmati Rice

Basmati rice is an aromatic long-grain rice that has a mild, nutlike flavor. It works well in salads and side dishes and as a stuffing base for pork or poultry dishes. This dish is a fine accompaniment for grilled or roasted poultry or seafood, including our Rotisserie-Style Roast Chicken (page 111), Apricot Grilled Pork Tenderloin (page 136), and Fiery Curry Tilapia (page 113).

1⅔ cups Homemade Vegetable Broth (page 68) or
    reduced-sodium, low-fat vegetable broth
¾ cup basmati rice
2 tablespoons finely chopped carrots
Pinch salt
¼ teaspoon ground cumin
¼ teaspoon ground cinnamon
⅛ teaspoon curry powder

Bring the vegetable broth to a boil. Stir in the rice, carrots, and seasonings and reduce heat to low. Cover and simmer for 15 to 20 minutes, or until all the water is absorbed and the rice is tender. Serve hot.

Yield: 4 servings

**Nutritional Information
Per Serving (¼ of recipe):**

Calories: 138
Fat: 0.3 g
  Saturated Fat: 0 g
  Monounsaturated Fat: 0.1 g
  Polyunsaturated Fat: 0.1 g
Cholesterol: 0 g
Sodium: 2 mg
Carbohydrate: 31.4 g
Dietary Fiber: 1.3 g
Sugars: 0.2 g
Starches: 29.5 g
Protein: 3.1 g
Diabetic Exchanges:
  2 Starch/Bread

Wild Rice Porcini

The porcini mushroom, also known as the cèpe mushroom, is considered by many to be the finest tasting variety of wild mushroom. Fresh porcini mushrooms can be difficult to find in supermarkets, mainly because of their cost and relatively short shelf life. Dried porcini are readily available and work quite well in dishes such as this one.

¾ cup wild rice
Canola cooking spray
1 teaspoon olive oil
¼ cup chopped yellow onion
1 cup reconstituted dried porcini mushrooms,
    drained and chopped
1 clove garlic, minced
1 tablespoon minced fresh parsley, or 1 teaspoon
    dried parsley flakes
¼ cup Homemade Chicken Broth (page 66) or
    reduced-sodium, low-fat chicken broth
Dash ground black pepper

Yield: 4 servings

**Nutritional Information
Per Serving (¼ of recipe):**

Calories: 110
Fat: 1.5 g
  Saturated Fat: 0.2 g
  Monounsaturated Fat: 0.9 g
  Polyunsaturated Fat: 0.3 g
Cholesterol: 0 g
Sodium: 5 mg
Carbohydrate: 21.7 g
Dietary Fiber: 2.2 g
Sugars: 0.3 g
Starches: 2.3 g
Protein: 3.9 g
Diabetic Exchanges:
  1 Starch/Bread, 1 Vegetable,
  ½ Fat

Cook wild rice according to package directions.

Heat a large nonstick skillet over medium heat. Away from the heat source, spray with cooking spray and add the oil. Return to the heat and sauté the onion until it softens, about 5 minutes. Add the mushrooms and sauté for 2 minutes. Add the garlic and parsley and sauté for 1 minute. Add the broth, pepper, and cooked wild rice and simmer for 5 minutes, or until heated through, stirring occasionally. Serve hot.

Lemon Couscous

Couscous is a type of pasta made from granules of semolina that have been precooked and dried. It is ridiculously easy to prepare, requiring only that you add it to boiling water and let it sit for a few minutes, covered. It is well suited for salads, side dishes, and stews and can be seasoned in an endless number of ways. If you wish, you can substitute orange juice and orange zest for the lemon in this recipe.

2 cups plus 2 tablespoons water
2 tablespoons lemon juice
1/3 cup thinly sliced scallions
1 1/3 cups couscous, uncooked
2 teaspoons grated lemon zest

Bring the water and lemon juice to a boil in a medium saucepan. Add the scallions, then remove from the heat. Stir in the couscous and lemon zest. Cover and let stand for 5 minutes, or until the liquid has been absorbed and the couscous is tender. Fluff the couscous with a fork and serve.

Yield: 8 servings, about 1/2 cup per serving

Nutritional Information Per Serving (1/2 cup):

Calories: 110
Fat: 0.2 g
  Saturated Fat: 0 g
  Monounsaturated Fat: 0 g
  Polyunsaturated Fat: 0.1 g
Cholesterol: 0 g
Sodium: 6 mg
Carbohydrate: 22.9 g
Dietary Fiber: 1.6 g
Sugars: 0.1 g
Starches: 0.1 g
Protein: 3.8 g
Diabetic Exchanges:
  1 1/2 Starch/Bread

Whole Wheat Irish Soda Bread

This flavorful, slightly dense bread tastes as good the next day as it does fresh-baked. Sliced and toasted leftovers are a breakfast bonus. If you do not like the flavor of caraway seeds, you can leave them out of this recipe and still have a great loaf of bread.

2 cups unbleached all-purpose flour
2 cups whole wheat flour
2 tablespoons sugar
2 teaspoons baking soda
½ teaspoon salt
3 tablespoons light margarine, softened
¼ cup golden raisins or currants
½ cup dark raisins
1 teaspoon caraway seeds, optional
1½ cups plus 1 tablespoon low-fat buttermilk

Preheat oven to 350 degrees F. Line a baking sheet with parchment paper.

In a large bowl, combine the flours, sugar, baking soda, and salt. Cut in the margarine until it is incorporated. Stir in the raisins and caraway seeds, if desired. Add the buttermilk and work into the flour mixture with a rubber spatula until the liquid is absorbed. Shape the dough into a ball with your hands and place on a floured surface. Knead the dough for about 1 minute, then shape into a round loaf about 3½ inches high. Cut a ½-inch-deep X into the top of the loaf (cuts should be about 2½ inches long).

Place the loaf on the baking sheet and bake for 45 minutes. Remove to a wire rack to cool.

Yield: 1 loaf, 16 slices

Nutritional Information Per Serving (1 slice):

Calories: 153
Fat: 1.8 g
  Saturated Fat: 0.4 g
  Monounsaturated Fat: 0.5 g
  Polyunsaturated Fat: 0.6 g
Cholesterol: 1 g
Sodium: 271 mg
Carbohydrate: 30.9 g
Dietary Fiber: 2.5 g
Sugars: 5.6 g
Starches: 0.4 g
Protein: 4.7 g
Diabetic Exchanges:
  2 Starch/Bread

9

Desserts and Snacks

Toasted Almond Biscotti

Cranberry-Orange Biscotti

Chocolate Peanut Cookies

Moist and Chewy Peanut Butter Cookies

Stovetop Rice Pudding

Down-Home Bread Pudding

Aunt Christine's Banana Bread

Chocolate Chip Banana Bread

Georgia Peach Pie

Banana Cream Pie

Chocolate Coconut Cream Pie

Apple Blueberry Cobbler

Key Lime Cheesecake Squares

Hazelnut Chocolate Cheesecake

Baklava

Frozen Hot Chocolate

Baked Apples with Walnuts and Raisins

Chocolate-Covered Sunshine Treats

Summer Fruit Salad

Broiled Peaches with Raspberry Cream

Cherry Applesauce

Caribbean Coconut-Laced Plantain

Peach Beach Yogurt Pops

Fried Ice Cream with Raspberry Cream Sauce

Mardi Gras Popcorn

Fruit-Nut Trail Mix

In this age of supersizing, dessert has been transformed from a sweet treat at the end of a meal to a sweet feast that can contain more calories, fat, and carbohydrate than the rest of the meal combined. Dessert is meant to please the palate and to send a friendly reminder to your brain that the meal is over. It shouldn't be something that pushes you over the edge, from being satisfied to being stuffed. Like appetizers, desserts are not needed at every meal. Then again, a little dessert can bring a happy ending to a good dinner, and an assortment of desserts is a nice offering when entertaining guests.

You may have heard the saying that there are no bad foods. Well, that's also true for desserts, provided you pay attention to serving size and make appropriate choices based on your meal plan. We have included a variety of desserts to suit different needs, from quick and easy sweet-tooth pleasers to more elegant delicacies, and we created them so they can be incorporated into most meal plans.

We do not rely heavily on sugar in our recipes, including our desserts, preferring instead to use fruit, naturally sweet foods, and other sweeteners. However, the American Diabetes Association has modified its nutritional recommendations regarding the use of sucrose (table sugar) as part of a diabetic diet. It now says that "scientific evidence has shown that the use of sucrose as part of the meal plan does not impair blood glucose control in individuals with type 1 or type 2 diabetes." It goes on to say "You need to work sugar into the meal plan that you have set up with your dietitian. Sugar is not a 'free food.' It counts as a carbohydrate. When you choose to eat foods that contain sugar, you need to substitute them for carbohydrate foods in your meal plan."

Looking for something special to serve? Try our Caribbean Coconut-Laced Plantain, Broiled Peaches with Raspberry Cream, or Hazelnut Chocolate Cheesecake. Want something easy to make that you and your kids can enjoy? Try our Peach Beach Pops, Frozen Hot Chocolate, or Cherry Applesauce. How about something for a casual party or get-together? Whip up some Key Lime Cheesecake Squares or Chocolate-Covered Sunshine Treats, both of which can be made ahead of time and kept in the refrigerator. How about baking something with an aroma that will carry throughout the house? Both our Toasted Almond Biscotti and Cranberry-Orange Biscotti fit the bill, as does Aunt Christine's Banana Bread, Apple Blueberry Cobbler, and Georgia Peach Pie. We've also included some comfort foods to satisfy your soul, including Down-Home Bread Pudding, Stovetop Rice Pudding, and Moist and Chewy Peanut Butter Cookies.

Snacks are a bit different. On one hand, regularly scheduled snacks are an important component of meal planning, helping with the overall goal of diabetes management in keeping blood sugar levels as balanced as possible throughout the day. On the other hand, uncontrolled snacking or eating inappropriate snacks can negatively affect a meal plan and blood sugar levels. It's a bit of a double-edged sword because you need to include snacks in your daily routine, but it's far too easy to snack on the wrong foods. Free foods, such as celery sticks, make good munchies because they have less of an impact on sugar levels and meal plans. They usually don't need to be counted in meal planning when eaten in small amounts throughout the course of the day.

Toasted Almond Biscotti

Biscotti were originally created by an Italian baker and were flavored with almonds, which were a widely available commodity at the time. This recipe for a delicious, low-fat version of the traditional, classic style of biscotti contains no added sugar.

½ cup Splenda Granular
2 tablespoons light margarine
4 egg whites, lightly beaten
2 teaspoons almond extract
2 cups all-purpose flour
2 teaspoons baking powder
¼ teaspoon salt
¼ cup finely chopped toasted almonds
2 tablespoons sliced almonds

**Yield: 30 servings,
1 biscotti per serving**

**Nutritional Information
Per Serving (1 biscotti):**

Calories: 55
Fat: 2.2 g
  Saturated Fat: 0.2 g
  Monounsaturated Fat: 1.3 g
  Polyunsaturated Fat: 0.5 g
Cholesterol: 0 mg
Sodium: 79 mg
Carbohydrate: 7 g
Dietary Fiber: 0.6 g
Sugars: 0 g
Starches: 0.1 g
Protein: 2 g
Diabetic Exchanges:
  ½ Starch/Bread, ½ Fat

Preheat oven to 375 degrees F.

In a medium bowl, beat the Splenda and margarine with an electric mixer. Add the egg whites and almond extract and mix well.

In a large bowl, combine the flour, baking powder, and salt. Mix in the egg mixture and the chopped almonds.

Form the dough into a ball and cut in half. Roll each half into a 12-inch log, then flatten each log until it is 2½ inches wide. Sprinkle and press lightly into each loaf 1 tablespoon sliced almonds. Place each loaf on a nonstick baking sheet and bake for 20 minutes, or until the outside of the loaf becomes golden. Remove the loaves to a large cutting board; when cool enough to handle, slice each loaf into 15 ¾-inch-thick slices.

Return the sliced biscotti to the baking sheet and bake for 10 minutes. Flip the slices and bake for another 5 to 7 minutes, or until golden.

Serve the biscotti warm or store them in an airtight container once they are completely cooled. Putting warm biscotti in a sealed container will affect their crispness and texture.

Cranberry-Orange Biscotti

Sweet morsels of dried fruit are scattered throughout crunchy biscotti to create a colorful and delightful treat that is especially well suited for the holiday season.

2¼ cups all-purpose flour
1½ teaspoons baking powder
Pinch salt
½ cup margarine
¼ cup light brown sugar
2 eggs
1 teaspoon pure vanilla extract
2 tablespoons minced orange zest
¼ cup minced dried cranberries

Preheat oven to 375 degrees F.

In a large bowl, mix together the flour, baking powder, and salt.

In another bowl, beat the margarine and sugar until creamy, about 2 minutes. Beat in the eggs and vanilla extract. Stir in the flour mixture, orange zest, and cranberries.

Form the dough into a ball and cut in half. Roll each half into a 15-inch log, then flatten each log until it is 2½ inches wide. Place each flattened loaf on a nonstick baking sheet and bake for 20 minutes, or until golden. Remove the loaves to a large cutting board; when cool enough to handle, slice each loaf into 18 ¾-inch-thick slices.

Return the sliced biscotti to the baking sheet and bake for 10 minutes. Flip the slices and bake for another 10 minutes, or until the biscotti turn golden.

Serve the biscotti warm or store them in an airtight container once they are completely cooled. Putting warm biscotti in a sealed container will affect their crispness and texture.

Yield: 36 servings, 1 biscotti per serving

Nutritional Information Per Serving (1 biscotti):

Calories: 65
Fat: 2.9 g
  Saturated Fat: 0.6 g
  Monounsaturated Fat: 1.3 g
  Polyunsaturated Fat: 0.9 g
Cholesterol: 12 mg
Sodium: 49 mg
Carbohydrate: 8.3 g
Dietary Fiber: 0.3 g
Sugars: 2.1 g
Starches: 0.1 g
Protein: 1.2 g
Diabetic Exchanges:
  ½ Starch/Bread, ½ Fat

Chocolate Peanut Cookies

The classic combination of chocolate and peanuts team up once again for a light and crunchy cookie that is low in fat and carbohydrate.

2 egg whites
1 cup Splenda Granular
6 tablespoons unsweetened cocoa powder, sifted
1½ cups coarsely ground peanuts

Preheat oven to 325 degrees F.

Beat the egg whites with an electric mixer until stiff, using a whisk attachment at high speed. Reduce speed to medium and slowly add the Splenda and cocoa. Beat until thick, about 3 minutes. Remove bowl from mixer and fold in the peanuts with a rubber spatula until mixed.

Place the cookie dough in tablespoon-size portions on a nonstick baking sheet with at least 2 inches between them. Bake for 15 minutes, or until cookies are crisp. Transfer to a wire rack and cool.

**Yield: 30 servings,
1 cookie per serving**

**Nutritional Information
Per Serving (1 cookie):**

Calories: 46
Fat: 3.8 g
  Saturated Fat: 0.5 g
  Monounsaturated Fat: 1.8 g
  Polyunsaturated Fat: 1.2 g
Cholesterol: 0 mg
Sodium: 4 mg
Carbohydrate: 2.2 g
Dietary Fiber: 0.9 g
Sugars: 0.1 g
Starches: 0.5 g
Protein: 2.2 g
Diabetic Exchanges:
  ½ Starch/Bread, ½ Fat

Moist and Chewy Peanut Butter Cookies

These chewy peanut butter cookies aren't loaded with fat or cholesterol and they are simple to make. If you prefer crisper cookies, bake for an additional 3 minutes. You can store these in a resealable plastic bag or container for a few days once they have cooled completely.

¾ cup all-purpose flour
¼ cup whole wheat flour
1 teaspoon baking powder
1 tablespoon orange juice
2 tablespoons water
1 tablespoon unsweetened applesauce
½ teaspoon pure vanilla extract
1 egg white
¼ cup light margarine
2 teaspoons granulated sugar
3 tablespoons reduced-fat creamy peanut butter

**Yield: 12 servings,
1 cookie per serving**

**Nutritional Information
Per Serving (1 cookie):**

Calories: 82
Fat: 3.5 g
  Saturated Fat: 0.7 g
  Monounsaturated Fat: 1.3 g
  Polyunsaturated Fat: 1.1 g
Cholesterol: 0 mg
Sodium: 83 mg
Carbohydrate: 10.7 g
Dietary Fiber: 0.8 g
Sugars: 1.6 g
Starches: 0.9 g
Protein: 2.5 g
Diabetic Exchanges:
  ½ Starch/Bread, 1 Fat

Combine all ingredients in a large bowl. Cover with plastic wrap and refrigerate for 3 hours.

Preheat oven to 350 degrees F.

Roll the chilled dough into 12 balls and place on a nonstick baking sheet, spaced at least 2 inches apart. Press each ball down with the tines of a fork facing one direction, then press down again a half-turn around to form a criss-cross pattern. Bake for 12 minutes, or until just crisp around the edges. Cool on a wire rack.

Stovetop Rice Pudding

This sweet and creamy version of rice pudding can be prepared quickly in a saucepan and is delicious served either warm or chilled. If you plan on serving it chilled, you may want to add 2 tablespoons skim milk during the last minute of cooking.

Yield: 6 servings

1 egg, beaten
1¾ cups skim milk, divided
½ teaspoon pure vanilla extract
¼ teaspoon ground cinnamon
¼ cup evaporated nonfat milk
2 tablespoons Splenda Granular
1½ cups cooked white rice
¼ teaspoon salt substitute
½ cup golden raisins

**Nutritional Information
Per Serving (¼ of recipe):**

Calories: 139
Fat: 1.1 g
　Saturated Fat: 0.3 g
　Monounsaturated Fat: 0.4 g
　Polyunsaturated Fat: 0.2 g
Cholesterol: 37 mg
Sodium: 54 mg
Carbohydrate: 27.1 g
Dietary Fiber: 0.7 g
Sugars: 11.5 g
Starches: 1.6 g
Protein: 5.4 g
Diabetic Exchanges:
　2 Starch/Bread

In a small bowl, mix the egg with ½ cup skim milk, vanilla, and cinnamon.

In a saucepan, combine 1¼ cups skim milk, evaporated milk, Splenda, cooked rice, and salt substitute. Cook over medium heat, stirring constantly, until the pudding thickens and becomes creamy.

Remove the saucepan from the heat and slowly pour the egg-milk mixture into it, stirring quickly. Stir in the raisins and return to the heat. Cook for another 2 to 3 minutes, stirring constantly, until the pudding thickens and the raisins plump up a little bit. Serve warm or cover and refrigerate until chilled.

Down-Home Bread Pudding

Hints of vanilla and cinnamon flavor this moist bread pudding that gets added sweetness and texture from raisins and dates. It is simple to prepare and is particularly nice during the autumn and winter months.

½ cup fat-free egg substitute
2¼ cups skim milk
1 teaspoon pure vanilla extract
½ teaspoon ground cinnamon
¼ teaspoon salt substitute
1 tablespoon brown sugar
7 slices reduced-calorie white bread, cut into 1-inch cubes (about 2 cups)
2 tablespoons chopped dates
6 tablespoons raisins
Canola cooking spray

Yield: 6 servings

**Nutritional Information
Per Serving (⅙ of recipe):**

Calories: 167
Fat: 1.2 g
  Saturated Fat: 0.2 g
  Monounsaturated Fat: 0.3 g
  Polyunsaturated Fat: 0.4 g
Cholesterol: 2 mg
Sodium: 251 mg
Carbohydrate: 31.3 g
Dietary Fiber: 1.5 g
Sugars: 12.5 g
Starches: 1.5 g
Protein: 8 g
Diabetic Exchanges:
  2 Starch/Bread

Preheat oven to 350 degrees F.

In a large bowl, combine the egg substitute, milk, vanilla, cinnamon, salt substitute, and brown sugar. Add the bread cubes, dates, and raisins and stir until combined.

Spray a 1½-quart baking dish with cooking spray and pour the bread pudding mixture into it. Set the baking dish in a pan with 1 inch of hot water in it and set the pan on the middle rack of the oven. Bake for 45 minutes, or until a toothpick inserted into the middle of the pudding comes out clean. Serve warm.

Aunt Christine's Banana Bread

Bananas and applesauce help create a moist fresh-baked bread that no one will ever guess is so low in fat. Not only does this taste delicious fresh, but it can also be frozen (wrap well in plastic wrap and foil). If you like, add ¼ cup chopped walnuts to the dry ingredients.

Yield: 1 loaf, 12 servings

⅓ cup unsweetened applesauce
¼ cup granulated sugar
1 egg
2 egg whites
1⅓ cups all-purpose flour
1 teaspoon baking powder
¼ teaspoon baking soda
½ teaspoon salt
1 cup mashed very ripe banana (about 2 small bananas)
Canola cooking spray

Nutritional Information Per Serving (1 slice):

Calories: 95
Fat: 0.6 g
  Saturated Fat: 0.2 g
  Monounsaturated Fat: 0.2 g
  Polyunsaturated Fat: 0.1 g
Cholesterol: 18 mg
Sodium: 71 mg
Carbohydrate: 19.9 g
Dietary Fiber: 0.9 g
Sugars: 4.7 g
Starches: 0.1 g
Protein: 2.7 g
Diabetic Exchanges:
  1 Starch/Bread

Preheat oven to 350 degrees F.

In a large bowl, mix the applesauce and sugar. Add the egg and egg whites and beat well.

In another bowl, combine the dry ingredients, then stir into the applesauce mixture. Add the mashed bananas and mix well.

Spray a 9-by-5-inch loaf pan with cooking spray. Spread the bread batter evenly in the pan and bake for 40 to 45 minutes, or until a toothpick inserted in the center comes out clean. Serve warm, or cool completely and wrap in plastic wrap until ready to serve.

Chocolate Chip Banana Bread

Fluffy whole wheat banana bread comes together with just the right amount of chocolate chips for a moist, low-fat bread that makes an exceptional treat.

Yield: 1 loaf, 16 servings

¾ cup mashed ripe or overripe banana (about 2 small bananas)
2 tablespoons granulated sugar
⅓ cup unsweetened applesauce
¼ cup plain nonfat yogurt
2 egg whites
½ teaspoon pure vanilla extract
¾ cup all-purpose flour
¼ cup whole wheat flour
1 teaspoon baking powder
1 teaspoon baking soda
½ cup semisweet chocolate chips
Canola cooking spray

**Nutritional Information
Per Serving (¹⁄₁₆ of recipe):**

Calories: 84
Fat: 2.3 g
  Saturated Fat: 1.3 g
  Monounsaturated Fat: 0.7 g
  Polyunsaturated Fat: 0.1 g
Cholesterol: 0 mg
Sodium: 112 mg
Carbohydrate: 15.3 g
Dietary Fiber: 1.1 g
Sugars: 6.3 g
Starches: 0.2 g
Protein: 1.9 g
Diabetic Exchanges:
  1 Starch/Bread, ½ Fat

Preheat oven to 350 degrees F.

In a large bowl, combine the banana, sugar, applesauce, yogurt, egg whites, and vanilla.

In another bowl, combine the flours, baking powder, and baking soda. Stir into the banana mixture. Add the chocolate chips and stir until well combined.

Pour the batter into a 9-by-5-inch loaf pan that has been sprayed with cooking spray. Bake for 30 to 35 minutes, or until a toothpick inserted in the center comes out clean.

Georgia Peach Pie

Farm-fresh peaches are touched with a hint of almond, baked in a reduced-fat pie crust, and topped with whipped topping for a summertime treat not to be ignored. If you've never had fresh peach pie, now is your chance.

About 2½ pounds fresh peaches
2½ tablespoons fresh lemon juice
1 tablespoon Splenda Granular
3 tablespoons cornstarch
⅛ teaspoon almond extract
⅛ teaspoon salt substitute
1 reduced-fat pie crust for a two-crust 9-inch pie
2 teaspoons skim milk
Fat-free nondairy whipped topping, optional

Position a rack in the lower half of the oven and preheat oven to 425 degrees F.

Peel and pit peaches, and cut into ¼-inch-thick slices; you should have 5 cups of peaches. Combine peaches with lemon juice, Splenda, cornstarch, almond extract, and salt substitute. Let the pie filling stand for about 15 minutes, stirring occasionally.

Line a 9-inch pie pan with the bottom crust. Pour the peach filling into the pie crust (if there is too much liquid, use a slotted spoon). Use your finger to dot the overhanging edge of the bottom pie crust with cold water. Cover the pie with the top crust and seal the edges of the pie crust together, crimping with your fingers. Use a paring knife to cut 4 evenly spaced steam vents in the top of the crust.

Lightly brush the top pie crust with skim milk. Use just enough to moisten the top crust, so do not brush excessively or allow any milk to puddle. Bake for 25 minutes.

Remove the pie from oven, set on a baking sheet, and return to the oven. Reduce the temperature to 350 degrees F., and bake until juices begin to bubble though the steam vents and the crust becomes golden, about 35 to 40 minutes.

Yield: 8 servings

**Nutritional Information
Per Serving (1 slice):**

Calories: 239
Fat: 10.6 g
  Saturated Fat: 2.3 g
  Monounsaturated Fat: 4.5 g
  Polyunsaturated Fat: 0 g
Cholesterol: 0 mg
Sodium: 189 mg
Carbohydrate: 35.9 g
Dietary Fiber: 2.2 g
Sugars: 3.2 g
Starches: 0.2 g
Protein: 3.8 g
Diabetic Exchanges:
  1 Starch/Bread, 1½ Fruit,
  2 Fat

Remove the pie to a cooling rack and allow it to cool before serving. It is best to wait at least an hour before cutting. If you try to cut it while it is still hot, you will end up with messy, runny, leaking pieces of peach pie, and you will surely be disappointed.

Serve with 1 tablespoon of reduced-fat or reduced-calorie whipped topping on top of each piece, if desired.

Banana Cream Pie

This rendition of the decades-old favorite uses sugar-free pudding and fresh bananas to make a creamy, flavorful pie that everyone will enjoy.

Yield: 8 servings

1 9-inch reduced-fat pie shell
2 boxes instant sugar-free vanilla pudding
Fat-free skim milk, as required for pudding mix
1 teaspoon banana extract
2 large bananas, sliced
Fat-free nondairy whipped topping

Nutritional Information Per Serving (1 slice):

Calories: 219
Fat: 7.4 g
  Saturated Fat: 1.6 g
  Monounsaturated Fat: 3.1 g
  Polyunsaturated Fat: 0 g
Cholesterol: 2 mg
Sodium: 518 mg
Carbohydrate: 33.9 g
Dietary Fiber: 0.8 g
Sugars: 7.4 g
Starches: 0.5 g
Protein: 6.6 g
Diabetic Exchanges: 1½ Fruit, 1 Fat-Free Milk, 1 Fat

Preheat oven to 350 degrees F.

Bake the pie shell for 25 minutes, or until golden brown. Remove from oven and set aside.

Meanwhile, prepare the pudding according to package directions for pie filling, using fat-free milk. Whisk in the banana extract along with the milk.

Spread a ½-inch layer of pudding into the pie crust. Top with a layer of banana slices and cover with ½-inch pudding. Repeat with the remaining banana slices and top with remaining pudding.

Refrigerate for 2 hours, or until firm enough to cut. If the pudding does not seem firm enough to hold its shape when the pie is cut, put the entire pie in the freezer for an hour or two. Cut the pie into 8 equal portions and top each with 1 tablespoon whipped topping.

Chocolate Coconut Cream Pie

Chocolate pudding is laced with coconut, topped with a layer of whipped topping, and sprinkled with toasted coconut flakes for a rich, sweet treat with less than 24 grams of carbohydrate.

Yield: 8 servings

1 9-inch reduced-fat pie shell
2 boxes instant sugar-free chocolate pudding
Fat-free skim milk, as required for pudding mix
1½ teaspoons coconut extract
1 cup fat-free nondairy whipped topping
3 tablespoons unsweetened coconut flakes, toasted in oven

Preheat oven to 350 degrees F.

Bake the pie shell for 25 minutes, or until golden brown. Remove from oven and set aside.

Meanwhile, prepare the pudding, using fat-free milk, according to package directions for pie filling. Whisk in the coconut extract along with the milk.

Spoon the pudding into the pie crust and refrigerate until firm. Remove from refrigerator and top with the whipped topping, smoothing it out into a thin layer. Freeze for 2 hours, or until the whipped topping becomes a little dense and sticky.

Sprinkle the coconut flakes over the pie; cut into 8 equal pieces and serve.

**Nutritional Information
Per Serving (1 slice):**

Calories: 193
Fat: 8.6 g
  Saturated Fat: 2.8 g
  Monounsaturated Fat: 3.1 g
  Polyunsaturated Fat: 0 g
Cholesterol: 2 mg
Sodium: 194 mg
Carbohydrate: 23.5 g
Dietary Fiber: 0.4 g
Sugars: 8.5 g
Starches: 0.6 g
Protein: 6.5 g
Diabetic Exchanges:
  1 Starch/Bread, ½ Fat-Free Milk, 1½ Fat

Apple Blueberry Cobbler

Fresh apples and blueberries are covered with a thick layer of batter and baked, resulting in a moist, fluffy crust bubbling with warm, juicy fruit. Top with a dollop of fat-free whipped topping, if desired.

Canola cooking spray
4 cups thinly sliced peeled apples (about 1½ pounds medium apples)
½ cup fresh blueberries
2 teaspoons granulated sugar
½ teaspoon ground cinnamon
1 cup all-purpose flour, sifted
1 teaspoon baking powder
¼ teaspoon salt
2 egg whites, beaten
½ cup evaporated nonfat milk
3 tablespoons light margarine, melted

Yield: 8 servings

Nutritional Information Per Serving (1 slice):

Calories: 128
Fat: 1.9 g
  Saturated Fat: 0.3 g
  Monounsaturated Fat: 0.5 g
  Polyunsaturated Fat: 0.6 g
Cholesterol: 1 mg
Sodium: 170 mg
Carbohydrate: 24.8 g
Dietary Fiber: 2.2 g
Sugars: 1.8 g
Starches: 0.5 g
Protein: 3.9 g
Diabetic Exchanges: ½ Fruit, ½ Fat

Preheat oven to 325 degrees F. Lightly spray an 8-by-2-inch round nonstick cake pan with cooking spray.

Spread the apple slices evenly in the baking pan, then top with the blueberries.

In a small bowl, mix the sugar and cinnamon together. Sprinkle over the apple slices.

In a medium bowl, mix the flour, baking powder, and salt. Add the egg whites, milk, and margarine and mix until smooth. Pour the batter evenly over the fruit.

Bake for 55 minutes, or until a toothpick inserted into the top of the cobbler comes out clean. Remove from oven and cool on a rack for at least 20 minutes before serving. Serve warm.

Key Lime Cheesecake Squares

Great for a party, these low-fat, low-carbohydrate cheese-cake squares are just big enough to satisfy your sweet tooth. If you cannot find graham cracker crumbs, you can crush plain graham crackers easily by placing them in a resealable plastic bag and hitting them with the flat side of a meat mallet, or you can process them briefly in a food processor. If you cannot find lime extract, then try lemon extract instead for a lemon version and use lemon zest on top.

Canola cooking spray
²⁄₃ cup plain graham cracker crumbs
1 8-ounce package light cream cheese, softened
1 8-ounce package fat-free cream cheese, softened
1 cup part-skim ricotta cheese
¹⁄₃ cup granulated sugar
¹⁄₂ teaspoon pure vanilla extract
1 tablespoon lime extract
1 egg
4 egg whites
Fat-free nondairy whipped topping, optional
Thinly sliced lime zest, optional garnish

Preheat oven to 350 degrees F.

Coat a 13¹⁄₂-by-9¹⁄₂-by-2-inch baking pan with cooking spray. Sprinkle the cracker crumbs evenly in the bottom of the pan. Place a sheet of wax paper over the crumbs and press the crumbs down.

In a stand mixer set at medium speed, beat the cream cheeses, ricotta cheese, sugar, vanilla and lime extract until smooth. Add the egg and egg whites and beat well. Pour the batter into the pan over the graham cracker crumbs and even out with a rubber spatula.

Bake for 25 minutes, or until the cheesecake cracks a little bit around the edges and barely moves in the center when you shake the pan. Remove to a wire rack and cool for an hour. Cover with plastic wrap and refrigerate overnight.

Cut into 24 squares and serve each square with a teaspoon of fat-free whipped topping sprinkled with a few thin slices of lime zest, if desired.

Yield: 24 squares

**Nutritional Information
Per Serving (1 square):**

Calories: 63
Fat: 2.5 g
  Saturated Fat: 1.7 g
  Monounsaturated Fat: 0.8 g
  Polyunsaturated Fat: 0.1 g
Cholesterol: 21 mg
Sodium: 144 mg
Carbohydrate: 4.6 g
Dietary Fiber: 0 g
Sugars: 3.8 g
Starches: 0.6 g
Protein: 5.4 g
Diabetic Exchanges:
  ¹⁄₂ Starch/Bread, ¹⁄₂ Fat

Hazelnut Chocolate Cheesecake

Enjoy a luxurious ending to a meal with a slice of rich New York-style cheesecake laced with milk chocolate and hazelnut. You can substitute your favorite sugar-free strawberry or raspberry flavored syrup for the hazelnut syrup, if desired.

Yield: 12 servings

Nutritional Information Per Serving (¹⁄₁₂ of recipe):

Calories: 322
Fat: 15.9 g
  Saturated Fat: 8.6 g
  Monounsaturated Fat: 5.2 g
  Polyunsaturated Fat: 1.3 g
Cholesterol: 83 mg
Sodium: 652 mg
Carbohydrate: 26.7 g
Dietary Fiber: 1.3 g
Sugars: 22.5 g
Starches: 2.6 g
Protein: 19.8 g
Diabetic Exchanges: 2½ Low-Fat Milk, ½ Starch/Bread, 1 Fat

3⁄4 cup low-fat graham cracker crumbs
3 tablespoons light margarine, melted
Canola cooking spray
2 8-ounce packages light cream cheese, softened
2 8-ounce packages fat-free cream cheese, softened
¼ cup sugar
¼ cup Splenda Granular
1 teaspoon pure vanilla extract
6 ounces semisweet baking chocolate, melted
2 tablespoons sugar-free hazelnut syrup
2 eggs
4 egg whites

In a medium bowl, combine the cracker crumbs and margarine, stirring until well mixed. Coat the bottom of a 9-inch springform pan with cooking spray. Press the cracker mixture evenly into the bottom of the pan.

Preheat oven to 325 degrees F.

Beat the cream cheeses, sugar, Splenda, and vanilla until well blended. Mix in the melted chocolate, hazelnut syrup, eggs, and egg whites.

Pour the cake batter evenly over the crust and bake for 55 minutes, or until the center is almost set when you jiggle the pan. Remove from oven and run a knife around the rim of the pan to separate the cake from the sides of the pan. Cool on a wire rack, then remove the rim from the springform pan. Refrigerate overnight or until cold. Cut into 12 equal pieces and serve.

Baklava

We really pulled out all the stops trying to figure out a way to make a healthier version of this popular Greek pastry dripping in sugar and butter. You're going to be surprised at how good this turns out to be. Ground walnuts are surrounded by flaky phyllo dough and drenched in a sweetened honey syrup.

Yield: 6 servings, can be doubled

Nutritional Information Per Serving (⅙ of recipe):
Calories: 54
Fat: 1.6 g
  Saturated Fat: 0.2 g
  Monounsaturated Fat: 0.4 g
  Polyunsaturated Fat: 0.9 g
Cholesterol: 0 mg
Sodium: 66 mg
Carbohydrate: 8.5 g
Dietary Fiber: 0.4 g
Sugars: 0.3 g
Starches: 6.7 g
Protein: 1.3 g
Diabetic Exchanges: ½
  Starch/Bread, ½ Fat

For the Pastry:
2 tablespoons coarsely ground walnuts
¼ teaspoon ground cinnamon
1 teaspoon Splenda Granular
3 sheets phyllo dough, thawed
1 tablespoon light margarine, melted

For the Syrup:
½ cup water
1 tablespoon Splenda Granular
1 teaspoon pure honey
¾ teaspoon lemon juice

Preheat oven to 375 degrees F.

Prepare the pastry: Combine the walnuts, cinnamon, and Splenda in a small bowl.

Lay 1 phyllo sheet on a flat surface horizontally, so the longer side is facing you. Lightly brush with the margarine and lay the second sheet on top, lining up the edges. Lightly brush with the margarine and lay the third sheet on top, lining up the edges.

Still facing the long side of the layered phyllo, spoon the walnut mixture in a straight vertical line (away from you, not side to side) starting about 2 inches from the left-side edge. Spread the nut mixture until you have a 2½-inch-wide strip going the 12-inch length of the phyllo.

Fold the left-side edge of the sheets over to cover the nuts. Continue to fold, end over end, in 2½ inch widths, brushing lightly with the margarine every other time you make another fold, until you have one 2½-inch-by-12-inch roll of phyllo sheets. Brush the entire top and sides of the rolled pastry with the remaining margarine.

Lay out a piece of parchment paper and place the rolled pastry on it, buttered-side up. Using a pizza cutter, cut the roll into 6 slices diagonally on a 15 to 20 degree angle, without separating the slices from each other. Transfer the sliced roll, along with the parchment paper, to a baking sheet. Bake for 10 to 12 minutes, or until golden on the outside.

Meanwhile, prepare the syrup. Combine the water and Splenda in a small saucepan and heat over medium-high heat, stirring, until it starts to boil. Reduce heat to low and stir in the honey and lemon juice. Heat for 30 seconds, then remove from heat and set aside.

Remove the golden phyllo from the oven and slide onto a serving plate. Drizzle the warm syrup over and serve.

Frozen Hot Chocolate

This dessert delivers rich chocolate flavor with minimal calories, carbohydrate, or fat and is simple to prepare. Topped with whipped topping and shaved chocolate, it looks as good as it tastes.

Yield: 4 servings

3 cups ice
2 envelopes no-sugar-added hot cocoa mix
⅔ cup nonfat milk
⅓ cup evaporated skim milk
4 tablespoons fat-free nondairy whipped topping
1 teaspoon shaved semisweet chocolate

Process ice, cocoa mix, nonfat milk, and evaporated skim milk in a blender until smooth. Divide among 4 large wineglasses or dessert bowls. Top each serving with 1 tablespoon whipped topping and sprinkle with shaved chocolate. Serve immediately.

**Nutritional Information
Per Serving (¼ of recipe):**

Calories: 70
Fat: 0.6 g
  Saturated Fat: 0.3 g
  Monounsaturated Fat: 0.2 g
  Polyunsaturated Fat: 0 g
Cholesterol: 2 mg
Sodium: 121 mg
Carbohydrate: 10.6 g
Dietary Fiber: 0.4 g
Sugars: 7.5 g
Starches: 1.2 g
Protein: 5.2 g
Diabetic Exchanges: 1 Fat-Free
  Milk

Baked Apples with Walnuts and Raisins

Apples are stuffed with golden raisins and walnuts, baked until soft, and served with warm cinnamon-spiced cider spooned over. This is a great autumn dessert that is very simple to prepare.

Yield: 4 servings

- 1 tablespoon chopped walnuts
- 2 tablespoons golden raisins
- ½ cup apple cider
- ½ teaspoon ground cinnamon
- 4 small baking apples, unpeeled, washed, and cored
- 4 tablespoons fat-free nondairy whipped topping, optional

Nutritional Information Per Serving (1 apple):

Calories: 98
Fat: 1 g
  Saturated Fat: 0.1 g
  Monounsaturated Fat: 0.1 g
  Polyunsaturated Fat: 0.5 g
Cholesterol: 0 mg
Sodium: 2 mg
Carbohydrate: 24 g
Dietary Fiber: 3.3 g
Sugars: 13.3 g
Starches: 0 g
Protein: 0.5 g
Diabetic Exchanges: 1½ Fruit

Preheat oven to 375 degrees F.

In a small bowl, mix the walnuts and raisins together.

In another small bowl, mix the cider and cinnamon together.

Pare a strip of peel from around the top of each apple and discard. Stuff each cored apple with walnut-raisin mixture, dividing it equally among the apples. Arrange the stuffed apples in an 8-inch round baking pan or casserole dish.

Spoon the cider mixture over the apples, cover with aluminum foil, and bake for 20 minutes. Remove the foil and use a spoon to baste the apples with the juice. Return to the oven and bake for another 20 minutes, or until the apples are tender. Serve warm with a tablespoon of whipped topping per apple, if desired.

Chocolate-Covered Sunshine Treats

Sweet dried plums and apricots are coated with chocolate and rolled in coconut and almonds to create small treats with big flavor. Easy and quick to make, these treats can be kept for about a week in the refrigerator and are great for a party. You can also substitute other types of chopped or ground nuts for the almonds, if you prefer.

1¼ cups toasted almonds, chopped
1¼ cups unsweetened coconut, toasted
12 ounces semisweet chocolate morsels
1 tablespoon evaporated skim milk
25 pitted dried plums
25 pitted dried apricots

Line a large plate with wax paper. Place the almonds in a medium bowl. Place the coconut in another medium bowl.

Place the chocolate in a microwave-safe container and microwave for about 30 seconds, or until the chocolate sweats and softens. Stir the chocolate until melted and just warm. If it has not melted enough to stir, return to the microwave and heat for 10 seconds and stir again. Repeat, if necessary, until melted. Do not overheat the chocolate. Stir in the evaporated skim milk.

Using a fork, dip a piece of fruit into the melted chocolate. Allow excess chocolate to drip off, then roll in either the almond or coconut topping.

Place each finished piece of fruit on the plate lined with wax paper. Do not pile them on top of each other. If the plate gets filled up, lay another piece of wax paper on top and start another layer.

Refrigerate for at least an hour before serving.

Yield: 50 1-piece servings

Nutritional Information Per Serving (1 piece):

Calories: 105
Fat: 7 g
  Saturated Fat: 3.8 g
  Monounsaturated Fat: 2.3 g
  Polyunsaturated Fat: 0.6 g
Cholesterol: 0 mg
Sodium: 34 mg
Carbohydrate: 11.1 g
Dietary Fiber: 1.3 g
Sugars: 5.6 g
Starches: 0.6 g
Protein: 1.6 g
Diabetic Exchanges: 1 Fruit, 1 Fat

Summer Fruit Salad

Citrus, banana, melon, grapes, and pineapple combine with fresh mint leaves and lime zest for a sweet and refreshing treat perfect for a hot summer day. You can also use this as a topping for grilled chicken or a firm fish such as swordfish.

Yield: 8 servings, about
¾ cup per serving

Nutritional Information
Per Serving (⅛ of recipe):

Calories: 85
Fat: 0.4 g
  Saturated Fat: 0.1 g
  Monounsaturated Fat: 0 g
  Polyunsaturated Fat: 0.1 g
Cholesterol: 0 mg
Sodium: 5 mg
Carbohydrate: 21.2 g
Dietary Fiber: 1.5 g
Sugars: 5.4 g
Starches: 0.4 g
Protein: 1.2 g
Diabetic Exchanges: 1½ Fruit

1 banana, peeled and sliced
¼ cup no-pulp orange juice concentrate, thawed
2 teaspoons fresh lime juice
1 cup red seedless grapes
1 cup green seedless grapes
1 11-ounce can mandarin orange segments, packed in juice or water, drained
1 cup cantaloupe balls
1 8-ounce can pineapple chunks, packed in water or juice, drained
1 tablespoon minced fresh mint leaves
½ teaspoon grated lime zest
Fat-free nondairy whipped topping, optional

In a large bowl, toss all the ingredients except the whipped topping until well combined. Keep chilled in the refrigerator, covered, until ready to serve. If you wish, you can top with 1 tablespoon whipped topping per serving.

Broiled Peaches with Raspberry Cream

Fresh peaches are broiled and topped with fresh raspberries and a delicious raspberry cream sauce laced with Cognac. This is remarkably easy to make and the final result is impressive. It tastes marvelous and looks even better. You can omit the brandy to make this an alcohol-free (or kid-friendly) dessert.

Canola cooking spray
3 tablespoons plus 4 teaspoons fat-free nondairy whipped topping, divided
⅓ cup evaporated nonfat milk
1 teaspoon Cognac or brandy
2 tablespoons seedless red raspberry spreadable fruit
2 large ripe peaches, washed, halved, pit removed
8 fresh red raspberries

Preheat broiler.

Line a broiler-safe baking dish with aluminum foil and spray lightly with cooking spray.

Whisk 3 tablespoons whipped topping, evaporated milk, brandy, and raspberry spreadable fruit in a small mixing bowl. Chill until ready to use.

Place the 4 peach halves in the baking dish, cut side up. Broil for 3 to 5 minutes, or until the fruit is hot and the top dries and becomes slightly crusted.

Place each roasted peach half, cut side up, in a large margarita glass or dessert plate and drizzle with 1 tablespoon of the chilled raspberry sauce. Spoon 1 teaspoon whipped topping into each peach pit cavity and place 2 raspberries into the whipped topping. Serve immediately while the peach is still warm.

Yield: 4 servings

Nutritional Information Per Serving (¼ of recipe):
Calories: 93
Fat: 0.2 g
  Saturated Fat: 0 g
  Monounsaturated Fat: 0.1g
  Polyunsaturated Fat: 0.1 g
Cholesterol: 1 mg
Sodium: 29 mg
Carbohydrate: 19.4 g
Dietary Fiber: 2.7 g
Sugars: 5.2 g
Starches: 0.9 g
Protein: 2.4 g
Diabetic Exchanges:
  ½ Starch/Bread, 1 Fruit

Cherry Applesauce

Fresh-picked apples are simmered with apple juice and cinnamon and combined with sweet cherries for a colorful twist on a simple classic. Here in Central New York, where we have the luxury of being surrounded by an abundance of apples, this recipe is a great way to wrap up a fun-filled day of local apple picking. You can also freeze this until slushy and serve ice cold.

4 fresh-picked Cortland or McIntosh apples, peeled, cored, and chopped (about 2 cups)
½ cup apple juice
Pinch ground cinnamon
½ cup pitted, halved Bing cherries (fresh or frozen)

In a 2-quart saucepan, heat the apples, juice, and cinnamon over medium-high heat until the mixture begins to boil. Reduce heat and simmer for 10 minutes, stirring often. Add the cherries and continue to simmer over low heat for 3 minutes. Serve warm or refrigerate, covered, and serve cold.

Yield: 4 servings, ½ cup per serving

Nutritional Information Per Serving (½ cup):
Calories: 114
Fat: 0.8 g
 Saturated Fat: 0.1 g
 Monounsaturated Fat: 0.1 g
 Polyunsaturated Fat: 0.2 g
Cholesterol: 0 mg
Sodium: 1 mg
Carbohydrate: 28.6 g
Dietary Fiber: 3.3 g
Sugars: 15.6 g
Starches: 3 g
Protein: 0.6 g
Diabetic Exchanges: 2 Fruit

Caribbean Coconut-Laced Plantain

Slices of plantain are sautéed until soft and browned, served in a warm coconut rum–laced cream sauce and topped with frozen vanilla yogurt, whipped topping, and toasted coconut. You can try this with banana slices if you can't find plantains. The texture and flavor will not be the same, but it will still be tasty. If you do not want to use coconut rum, you can use a few drops of coconut extract mixed with 1 tablespoon water instead.

1 tablespoon light margarine
1 large plantain, sliced diagonally into ¼-inch-thick slices
1 tablespoon coconut rum
¼ cup evaporated nonfat milk
4 teaspoons nonfat frozen vanilla yogurt
4 teaspoons fat-free nondairy whipped topping
1 teaspoon toasted coconut flakes

Yield: 4 servings

Nutritional Information Per Serving (¼ of recipe):
Calories: 89
Fat: 1 g
 Saturated Fat: 0.4 g
 Monounsaturated Fat: 0.2 g
 Polyunsaturated Fat: 0.2 g
Cholesterol: 0 mg
Sodium: 31 mg
Carbohydrate: 17.5 g
Dietary Fiber: 1.1 g
Sugars: 2.1 g
Starches: 0.7 g
Protein: 2 g
Diabetic Exchanges:
 ½ Starch/Bread, ½ Fruit

Melt the margarine in a large nonstick skillet over medium-high heat. Add the plantain slices one at a time, sliding each piece into the melted margarine. Sauté until golden brown, about 1½ to 2 minutes per side.

Add the coconut rum and the evaporated milk. Swirl around and heat until the sauce bubbles and thickens, coating the plantain slices. Using a slotted spatula, remove the plantain slices to 4 dessert plates, overlapping the slices in the middle of each plate (fan the slices).

Spoon any remaining sauce over the plantain slices. Top with 1 teaspoon frozen yogurt and 1 teaspoon whipped topping. Sprinkle with a few coconut flakes and serve immediately.

Peach Beach Yogurt Pops

A frozen blend of peaches, yogurt, and juice serve as a homemade summertime treat that is low in fat and calories. You can substitute just about any type of fruit in this recipe. Try it with blueberries, strawberries, or raspberries. Try to match the yogurt flavor with the type of frozen fruit you are using.

1 16-ounce package frozen no-sugar-added peaches, thawed
1 cup low-fat peach yogurt
½ cup apple juice
10 3-ounce paper cups
10 wooden spoons

Blend the peaches, yogurt, and apple juice in a food processor. Spoon the mixture into paper cups and center a wooden spoon into each cup. Freeze until firm, 3 to 4 hours. To serve, tear the cup away from the yogurt pop.

Yield: 10 servings

Nutritional Information Per Serving (1 pop):

Calories: 45
Fat: 0.3 g
 Saturated Fat: 0.2 g
 Monounsaturated Fat: 0.1 g
 Polyunsaturated Fat: 0 g
Cholesterol: 1 mg
Sodium: 14 mg
Carbohydrate: 9.9 g
Dietary Fiber: 0.8 g
Sugars: 7.3 g
Starches: 0.4 g
Protein: 1.2 g
Diabetic Exchanges: 1 Fat-Free Milk

Fried Ice Cream with Raspberry Cream Sauce

Frozen yogurt is coated with hot corn flakes and coconut and surrounded with raspberry cream sauce for a decadent dessert surprisingly low in fat and calories. This recipe can be doubled.

1 cup nonfat vanilla or chocolate frozen yogurt
1 tablespoon fat-free nondairy whipped topping
2 tablespoons nonfat milk
1 tablespoon seedless red raspberry spreadable fruit
1 cup corn flakes cereal
2 teaspoons dried, unsweetened coconut flakes

Individually wrap ½-cup portions of frozen yogurt in plastic wrap and shape into balls. Freeze for 1 to 2 hours, or until firm.

Meanwhile, whisk together the whipped topping, milk, and spreadable fruit. Cover and refrigerate until ready to use.

Once the wrapped frozen yogurt balls are firm, preheat oven to 400 degrees F.

Arrange the corn flakes and coconut flakes in a single layer on a nonstick baking sheet. Bake for 5 minutes, or until hot but not browned. Remove to a medium bowl and toss until well combined.

Unwrap the frozen yogurt balls and quickly roll each one in the hot corn flake and coconut flake mixture until well coated. Place each coated ball in a margarita glass or a large wine glass or on a dessert plate and spoon the raspberry cream sauce around it. Serve immediately.

Yield: 2 servings, 1 cup per serving

Nutritional Information Per Serving (½ of recipe):

Calories: 156
Fat: 1.3 g
  Saturated Fat: 1.1 g
  Monounsaturated Fat: 0.1 g
  Polyunsaturated Fat: 0 g
Cholesterol: 0 mg
Sodium: 129 mg
Carbohydrate: 31.8 g
Dietary Fiber: 0.6 g
Sugars: 18.3 g
Starches: 12.4 g
Protein: 4 g
Diabetic Exchanges:
  1 Starch/Bread, ½ Fruit,
  ½ Fat-Free Milk

Mardi Gras Popcorn

Hot, air-popped popcorn is tossed with a spicy Creole seasoning mix for a great party snack that has no salt or fat. Set this out at your next Superbowl party.

4 cups freshly air-popped popcorn
1½ teaspoons Creole Seasoning Mix (page 215)

In a large bowl, toss the Creole Seasoning Mix with the popcorn until popcorn is well coated. Serve while the popcorn is still fresh and hot.

Yield: 4 1-cup servings

**Nutritional Information
Per Serving (1 cup):**

Calories: 32
Fat: 0.4 g
 Saturated Fat: 0.1 g
 Monounsaturated Fat: 0.1 g
 Polyunsaturated Fat: 0.2 g
Cholesterol: 0 mg
Sodium: 0 mg
Carbohydrate: 6.5 g
Dietary Fiber: 1.3 g
Sugars: 0 g
Starches: 0 g
Protein: 1 g
Diabetic Exchanges:
 ½ Starch/Bread

Fruit-Nut Trail Mix

A variety of sweet dried fruit is mixed with oat and wheat cereals and sunflower seeds for a low-fat trail mix that can provide a definite energy boost. Without the sunflower seeds and peanuts, use it to top plain low-fat yogurt for a tasty breakfast or lunch parfait.

2 cups toasted oat cereal
1 cup Wheat Chex cereal
¼ cup dried cranberries
¼ cup dark seedless raisins
¼ cup dried cherries
2 tablespoons chopped dried dates
1 tablespoon unsalted dry-roasted peanuts
1 tablespoon toasted sliced almonds
1 teaspoon unsalted sunflower seeds

In a large bowl, combine all ingredients and toss well. Store in an airtight container for up to 3 weeks.

**Yield: About 3 cups, or
9 ⅓-cup servings**

**Nutritional Information
Per Serving (⅓ cup):**

Calories: 91
Fat: 1.9 g
 Saturated Fat: 0.2 g
 Monounsaturated Fat: 0.8 g
 Polyunsaturated Fat: 0.5 g
Cholesterol: 0 mg
Sodium: 99 mg
Carbohydrate: 17.9 g
Dietary Fiber: 1.8 g
Sugars: 7.3 g
Starches: 3.1 g
Protein: 1.8 g
Diabetic Exchanges:
 1 Starch/Bread

10

Sauces and Condiments

Nona's Italian Marinara Sauce

Festive Holiday Cranberry Sauce

Rocco's Pomodoro Sauce

Cajun Tartar Sauce

Savory Mushroom Gravy

Homemade Gravy

Tzatziki Sauce

Guacamole Sauce

Raspberry-Brandy Cream Sauce

Zesty Dipping Sauce

Simple Sour Cream and Dijon
Sauce

Creamy Creole Dip

Fat-Free Salsa

Lemon-Herb Marinade

Jalapeño-Lime Marinade

Herbed Pepper Rub

Creole Seasoning Mix

No-Salt Cajun Spice Mix

House Italian Dressing

Raspberry Vinaigrette

Chunky Blue Cheese Dressing

Honey Mustard Vinaigrette

It's been said that you can judge a restaurant by its
sauces. The quality and variety of sauces can set one restaurant apart
from another. Strip away the sauce and you're often left with the same
food underneath. While this isn't the fairest of assessments, there is a
certain level of truth to it.

Sauces can really turn something ordinary into something special. A
well-developed sauce can add flavor, moistness, and color to a dish
without overpowering the food it is meant to complement. Unfortunately, far too many sauces are loaded to the hilt with things like fat,

salt, sugar, and cholesterol. This makes them an unhealthy choice for everyone, but even more so for people with diabetes.

We've created some great sauces that can make ordinary meals extraordinary, and we did it with a close eye on the nutritional content to make it easier for you to include them in your meal plan. We use ingredients such as fruit, homemade broth, juice, yogurt, and vegetables as bases in many of our sauces. When oil is called for, we use olive oil or canola oil to reduce the amount of saturated fat, and we use it sparingly. We also rely on spices, herbs, and other ingredients to enhance the flavor instead of adding salt. You will also find dips, dressings, and condiments that are perfect for salads, finger foods, crudités and canapés, as well as rubs and marinades for vegetables, meats, poultry, or seafood.

You can use our sauces and condiments to replace those called for in recipes from other sources that may not be suitable for your meal plan. You can also use them to bring some excitement to basic dishes that you may normally prepare, such as baked fish or grilled chicken. Try our Savory Mushroom Gravy over sliced turkey, Mock Mashed Potatoes, or a serving of no-cholesterol egg noodles. Drizzle Raspberry-Brandy Cream Sauce over a serving of nonfat frozen yogurt, fresh fruit, or Aunt Christine's Banana Bread. The culinary possibilities presented by this collection of sauces and condiments are limited only by the imagination.

Nona's Italian Marinara Sauce

This light, fresh-tasting, full-flavored tomato sauce can be made ahead of time and frozen in small batches for later use. Simply defrost in the microwave or overnight in the refrigerator, then reheat in a saucepan. If a thicker consistency is desired, add another 6-ounce can of tomato paste.

1 teaspoon olive oil
1 large yellow onion, chopped
2 cups sliced carrots
2 cloves garlic, minced
1 6-ounce can low-sodium tomato paste
1 29-ounce can low-sodium tomato purée
10 14.5-ounce cans low-sodium whole peeled
   tomatoes
⅛ teaspoon ground black pepper
1 teaspoon dried parsley
¾ teaspoon no-salt Italian seasoning
¼ teaspoon crushed red pepper flakes, optional

Heat the oil in a large stockpot over medium heat. Add the onions and carrots and sauté until the onions are softened and golden, about 10 minutes. Add the garlic and sauté for 30 seconds. Add the tomato paste and tomato purée and stir well. Stir in the remaining ingredients and reduce the heat to medium-low as soon as the mixture begins to simmer. Simmer for 2 hours, stirring occasionally. Using a wooden spoon, break apart the tomatoes to release their juice and simmer for another hour. Remove from the heat and set aside for about 20 minutes.

Position a food mill over a similar-size stockpot. Spoon the cooked tomatoes and sauce ingredients into the food mill in small batches and process everything, including the vegetables. Return the milled sauce to the stove and return to a simmer over medium heat, adjusting the spices, if desired.

Yield: 36 ½-cup servings

**Nutritional Information
Per Serving (½ cup):**

Calories: 41
Fat: 0.4 g
  Saturated Fat: 0.0 g
  Monounsaturated Fat: 0.1 g
  Polyunsaturated Fat: 0.1 g
Cholesterol: 0 mg
Sodium: 52 mg
Carbohydrate: 9.3 g
Dietary Fiber: 2.2 g
Sugars: 1.6 g
Starches: 0.9 g
Protein: 1.8 g
Diabetic Exchanges:
  2 Vegetable

Festive Holiday Cranberry Sauce

Add a little zest to the holiday table. As an extra bonus, cranberries, like many berries, contain phytochemicals that are believed to help fight cancer. This flavorful cranberry sauce goes well with roast poultry or baked ham and can be kept, refrigerated, for up to 4 days.

1 pound fresh whole cranberries
1½ cups water
2 teaspoons orange zest
2 teaspoons lime zest
¼ teaspoon ground cinnamon
6 whole cloves
1 tablespoon bourbon or whiskey
1 tablespoon orange juice concentrate
1 cup Splenda Granular, or similar sweetener

In a large saucepan, bring cranberries, water, orange zest, lime zest, cinnamon, and cloves to a boil over medium-high heat. Reduce heat to medium-low and simmer for 5 to 7 minutes, or until the cranberries begin to split open. Add the bourbon, orange juice concentrate, and Splenda and simmer for 1 minute, stirring. Cover and refrigerate overnight or until well chilled.

Yield: 16 2-tablespoon servings

Nutritional Information Per Serving (2 tablespoons):

Calories: 17
Fat: 0.1 g
  Saturated Fat: 0 g
  Monounsaturated Fat: 0 g
  Polyunsaturated Fat: 0 g
Cholesterol: 0 g
Sodium: 1 mg
Carbohydrate: 3.7 g
Dietary Fiber: 1.2 g
Sugars: 2.4 g
Starches: 0.1 g
Protein: 0.1 g
Diabetic Exchanges: Free

Rocco's Pomodoro Sauce

This just might be the ultimate tomato sauce! It's quick and easy to make and you can use it for everything from pasta to French bread pizza. You can easily double it or add ingredients such as roasted red peppers, sautéed mushrooms, or hot peppers to it. If you want a thicker sauce, stir in some tomato paste. If Italian-style tomatoes are not available, use regular low-sodium whole peeled tomatoes instead and add 1 tablespoon chopped fresh basil or ½ teaspoon dried basil.

1 28-ounce can low-sodium whole peeled Italian-style tomatoes
¼ teaspoon dried no-salt Italian seasoning
¼ teaspoon dried parsley flakes
1 teaspoon dry red wine
1 to 2 cloves garlic, finely chopped
Pinch crushed red pepper flakes, or to taste
Pinch freshly ground black pepper, or to taste

In a medium saucepan, combine the tomatoes, Italian seasoning, parsley, red wine, garlic, red pepper flakes, and black pepper. Break the tomatoes up with a wooden spoon. If there is a basil leaf in the can of tomatoes, mince it and add to the saucepan.

Cook over medium heat for 5 to 7 minutes, stirring occasionally, or until thoroughly heated and simmering.

Yield: 8 ¼-cup servings

**Nutritional Information
Per Serving (¼ cup):**

Calories: 21
Fat: 0.1 g
  Saturated Fat: 0 g
  Monounsaturated Fat: 0 g
  Polyunsaturated Fat: 0.1 g
Cholesterol: 0 mg
Sodium: 11 mg
Carbohydrate: 4.8 g
Dietary Fiber: 1.1 g
Sugars: 0.2 g
Starches: 0 g
Protein: 1 g
Diabetic Exchanges: 1 Vegetable

Cajun Tartar Sauce

This is a spiced-up, fat-free version of the classic sauce made popular for accompanying fried seafood. If you want "regular" tartar sauce, just omit the Cajun Spice Mix. This sauce works well for dipping seafood cakes, as well as for spreading on sandwiches such as our Cornmeal-Coated Chicken Sandwich (page 146). It can be kept for up to 4 days in the refrigerator, covered.

½ cup fat-free mayonnaise
2 tablespoons diced pickles
½ teaspoon Dijon mustard
½ to ¾ teaspoon No-Salt Cajun Spice Mix (page 215)
1 teaspoon red wine vinegar
Pinch salt substitute

Combine all ingredients and stir until well blended. Cover and refrigerate until ready to use.

Yield: 8 1-tablespoon servings

Nutritional Information Per Serving (1 tablespoon):

Calories: 11
Fat: 0 g
  Saturated Fat: 0 g
  Monounsaturated Fat: 0 g
  Polyunsaturated Fat: 0 g
Cholesterol: 0 mg
Sodium: 142 mg
Carbohydrate: 2.2 g
Dietary Fiber: 0 g
Sugars: 0.9 g
Starches: 1.1 g
Protein: 0.3 g
Diabetic Exchanges: Free

Savory Mushroom Gravy

Toss with no-yolk egg noodles to create a side dish or entrée. Use to top roasted chicken, turkey, or beef. Spoon over grilled burgers or use to make a hot open-faced turkey or roast beef sandwich. This low-fat, low-sodium gravy has a lot of possibilities.

1 tablespoon cornstarch
1 tablespoon water
Canola cooking spray
1 pound white mushrooms, sliced
1¼ cups Homemade Beef Broth (page 67) or reduced-sodium, low-fat beef broth
¼ cup water
1 shallot, minced
1 teaspoon dried parsley flakes
½ teaspoon Worcestershire sauce
Freshly ground black pepper, to taste
1 tablespoon evaporated nonfat milk
½ cup water

In a small bowl, blend the cornstarch and water with a spoon until smooth.

Heat a large nonstick skillet over medium-high

Yield: 4 ¼-cup servings

Nutritional Information Per Serving (¼ cup):

Calories: 47
Fat: 0.5 g
  Saturated Fat: 0.1 g
  Monounsaturated Fat: 0.1 g
  Polyunsaturated Fat: 0.1 g
Cholesterol: 3 mg
Sodium: 27 mg
Carbohydrate: 7.6 g
Dietary Fiber: 1.3 g
Sugars: 0.1 g
Starches: 0 g
Protein: 4.2 g
Diabetic Exchanges:
  ½ Starch/Bread

heat. Away from the heat source, spray the skillet with cooking spray. Return to the heat and sauté mushrooms until soft and brown.

Add the broth, water, shallot, parsley, and Worcestershire sauce and bring to a boil.

Stir in the cornstarch mixture and reduce the heat to medium-low. Season with freshly ground black pepper and simmer for 15 minutes, or until thickened to a gravylike consistency. Stir in the evaporated nonfat milk and water. Continue to simmer until thickened to the consistency you desire.

Homemade Gravy

This rich-tasting, low-fat gravy is easy to prepare using either Homemade Chicken Broth or canned chicken or turkey broth. If you are not roasting a bird to use this sauce for, then use ¼ cup reduced-sodium chicken or turkey broth in place of the defatted juices.

¼ cup cornstarch
¼ cup water
4 cups Homemade Chicken Broth (page 66), or reduced-sodium chicken or turkey broth
¼ cup pan juices from cooked turkey or chicken, defatted (see Note)
⅛ teaspoon Gravy Master, optional
Freshly ground black pepper, to taste

In a small bowl, blend the cornstarch and water with a spoon until smooth.

In a large saucepan, bring the broth and pan juices to a boil over medium heat. Slowly pour the cornstarch mixture into the boiling broth, whisking constantly, until the gravy thickens to the consistency you prefer. Whisk in the Gravy Master, if desired, and season lightly with black pepper.

Note: To defat pan juices: Ladle drippings from a roasted turkey or chicken into a clear container. Refrigerate for 30 minutes, or until the fat solidifies at the top of the container. Skim the layer of fat off with a spoon and discard. The remaining liquid is the defatted pan juice.

Yield: About 16 ¼-cup servings

Nutritional Information Per Serving (¼ cup):

Calories: 13
Fat: 0.1 g
  Saturated Fat: 0 g
  Monounsaturated Fat: 0.1 g
  Polyunsaturated Fat: 0 g
Cholesterol: 1 mg
Sodium: 6 mg
Carbohydrate: 2.6 g
Dietary Fiber: 0.2 g
Sugars: 0.1 g
Starches: 0 g
Protein: 0.3 g
Diabetic Exchanges: Free

Tzatziki Sauce

This is a refreshing, creamy Greek sauce that complements Chicken Souvlaki Plate (page 102), Greek Gyros (page 135), grilled dishes, and salads. You can also use this as a dip for crudité or pita bread, but we suggest that you mince the cucumber if that is how you're going to serve it. Leave out the garlic for a milder version, if desired.

1½ cups plain low-fat yogurt
1 small cucumber, peeled, halved lengthwise,
    seeded, and diced (about ½ cup)
1 clove garlic, minced
Pinch black pepper
½ teaspoon dried dill weed

Combine all ingredients and refrigerate, covered, until ready to use. This sauce can be kept, refrigerated and covered, for 2 or 3 days.

Yield: 16 1-tablespoon servings

Nutritional Information Per Serving (1 tablespoon):
Calories: 15
Fat: 0.4
  Saturated Fat: 0.2
  Monounsaturated Fat: 0.1
  Polyunsaturated Fat: 0
Cholesterol: 2 mg
Sodium: 16 mg
Carbohydrate: 1.8 g
Dietary Fiber: 0 g
Sugars: 1.7 g
Starches: 0 g
Protein: 1.3 g
Diabetic Exchanges: Free

Guacamole Sauce

Yes, you can eat guacamole! Use this as a dip or a sauce to top everything from tacos to grilled chicken and seafood. Unlike most homemade guacamole, this will actually last for a couple of days in the refrigerator and is much lower in fat.

1 ripe avocado
¼ cup seeded, diced tomato
2 tablespoons chopped yellow onion
1 teaspoon chopped garlic
1 pickled jalapeño pepper ring, diced
Dash hot sauce
⅔ cup plain nonfat yogurt
Dash ground black pepper
1 tablespoon chopped fresh cilantro
1 teaspoon lime juice

Slice the avocado in half, remove the pit, and spoon the flesh into a blender or food processor. Add the tomato, onion, garlic, jalapeno, hot sauce, yogurt, black pepper, cilantro, and lime juice. Purée until smooth, about 30 seconds. Store in a sealed container and refrigerate until ready to use.

Yield: 8 1-tablespoon servings

Nutritional Information Per Serving (1 tablespoon):
Calories: 52
Fat: 3.8 g
  Saturated Fat: 0.6 g
  Monounsaturated Fat: 2.4 g
  Polyunsaturated Fat: 0.5 g
Cholesterol: 0 mg
Sodium: 21 mg
Carbohydrate: 3.8 g
Dietary Fiber: 1.3 g
Sugars: 1.6 g
Starches: 0 g
Protein: 1.7 g
Diabetic Exchanges:
  1 Vegetable, 1 Fat

Raspberry-Brandy Cream Sauce

This simple, yet luxurious, fat-free sauce can add flair to any number of desserts. Try it on fat-free frozen yogurt topped with a dollop of fat-free whipped cream. Mix it with fresh fruit and spoon it on top of a ladyfinger. Use your imagination!

3 tablespoons fat-free nondairy whipped topping
⅓ cup evaporated nonfat milk
1 teaspoons brandy or Cognac
2 tablespoons seedless red raspberry spreadable
    fruit

Whisk together all the ingredients in a small bowl. Cover and chill; whisk again briefly when ready to use.

Yield: 5 2-tablespoon servings

Nutritional Information Per Serving (2 tablespoons):

Calories: 23
Fat: 0 g
  Saturated Fat: 0 g
  Monounsaturated Fat: 0 g
  Polyunsaturated Fat: 0 g
Cholesterol: 0 mg
Sodium: 4 mg
Carbohydrate: 4.9 g
Dietary Fiber: 0.1 g
Sugars: 3.5 g
Starches: 0.7 g
Protein: 0.1 g
Diabetic Exchanges: ½ Fruit

Zesty Dipping Sauce

This creamy horseradish sauce is great as a dip for Sweet Potato Fries (page 167), Baked French Fries (page 168), and Baked Onion Rings (page 64). Try it on grilled vegetable sandwiches or as a dip for crudités. The clincher? It has no fat and barely any calories per serving.

4 tablespoons fat-free sour cream
2 tablespoons fat-free mayonnaise
1 tablespoon prepared cream-style horseradish
2 tablespoons ketchup
2 tablespoons skim milk
⅛ teaspoon paprika
Pinch salt substitute

In a small bowl, combine all the ingredients and stir until well blended. Cover with plastic wrap and chill for about an hour before using. This can be kept for up to 4 days, covered and refrigerated.

Yield: 11 1-tablespoon servings

Nutritional Information Per Serving (1 tablespoon):

Calories: 11
Fat: 0 g
Saturated Fat: 0 g
Monounsaturated Fat: 0 g
Polyunsaturated Fat: 0 g
Cholesterol: 0 mg
Sodium: 63 mg
Carbohydrate: 2.3 g
Dietary Fiber: 0.1 g
Sugars: 1 g
Starches: 0.8 g
Protein: 0.3
Diabetic Exchanges: Free

Simple Sour Cream and Dijon Sauce

The name says it all. This works well with seafood dishes, such as Salmon Cakes (page 58) or baked fish, and can even be heated slightly and used to top chicken or pork. For a thinner sauce, add a little dry white wine or skim milk.

¾ cup light sour cream
¼ cup Dijon mustard

In a small bowl, combine both ingredients. Chill, covered, until ready to use as a dip or topping.

Yield: 16 1-tablespoon servings

Nutritional Information Per Serving (1 tablespoon):

Calories: 19
Fat: 1.4 g
  Saturated Fat: 0.8 g
  Monounsaturated Fat: 0.4 g
  Polyunsaturated Fat: 0 g
Cholesterol: 4 mg
Sodium: 93 mg
Carbohydrate: 1.2 g
Dietary Fiber: 0 g
Sugars: 0.4 g
Starches: 0 g
Protein: 0.8 g
Diabetic Exchanges: ½ Fat

Creamy Creole Dip

This dip is great with chips and crudités, but it also works well as a topping for seafood dishes, such as poached salmon, grilled shrimp, and crab cakes, as well as our Cornmeal-Coated Chicken Sandwich (page 146). It can be kept for up to 4 days, covered and refrigerated.

½ cup sour cream
1 tablespoon fat-free mayonnaise
1 teaspoon Creole Seasoning Mix (page 215)
2 tablespoons minced scallion, green part only
½ teaspoon Dijon mustard
¼ teaspoon Worcestershire sauce

Combine all the ingredients. Cover and refrigerate until well chilled.

Yield: 16 1-tablespoon servings

Nutritional Information Per Serving (1 tablespoon):

Calories: 12
Fat: 0.8 g
  Saturated Fat: 0.5 g
  Monounsaturated Fat: 0.2 g
  Polyunsaturated Fat: 0 g
Cholesterol: 3 mg
Sodium: 17 mg
Carbohydrate: 0.9 g
Dietary Fiber: 0.1 g
Sugars: 0.1 g
Starches: 0.1 g
Protein: 0.3 g
Diabetic Exchanges: Free

Fat-Free Salsa

There are many fat-free salsas available, but their sodium content can be outrageous. Our fat-free, low-sodium version tastes great. Turn this into a southwest-style salsa by adding some black beans and corn kernels.

1 14.5-ounce can low-sodium chopped tomatoes
⅓ cup minced red onion
1 clove garlic, minced
1 tablespoon minced jalapeño pepper
1 tablespoon chopped fresh cilantro
1 tablespoon lime juice
½ teaspoon salt substitute
½ teaspoon freshly ground black pepper

Combine all the ingredients and refrigerate for at least 3 hours before serving. Adjust the heat to suit your taste.

Yield: About 2 cups, or 16 2-tablespoon servings

Nutritional Information Per Serving (2 tablespoons):

Calories: 7
Fat: 0.1 g
  Saturated Fat: 0 g
  Monounsaturated Fat: 0 g
  Polyunsaturated Fat: 0 g
Cholesterol: 1 g
Sodium: 4 mg
Carbohydrate: 1.7 g
Dietary Fiber: 0.4 g
Sugars: 0.1 g
Starches: 0 g
Protein: 0.3 g
Diabetic Exchanges: Free

Lemon-Herb Marinade

This sodium-free marinade works well for summertime cookouts using chicken, shrimp, or pork. Just marinate the meat or shrimp for 15 to 20 minutes and grill or roast until done.

½ cup freshly squeezed lemon juice
¼ teaspoon crushed red pepper flakes
½ teaspoon freshly ground black pepper
¼ teaspoon salt substitute
¼ cup olive oil
3 cloves garlic, crushed
1 tablespoon chopped fresh parsley
½ teaspoon dried oregano
½ teaspoon dried basil

Whisk together the lemon juice, red pepper flakes, black pepper, salt substitute, and oil. Stir in the garlic, parsley, oregano, and basil. Use right away or refrigerate for up to a week

Yield: 16 1-tablespoon servings

Nutritional Information Per Serving (1 tablespoon):

Calories: 33
Fat: 3.4 g
  Saturated Fat: 0.5 g
  Monounsaturated Fat: 2.5 g
  Polyunsaturated Fat: 0.3 g
Cholesterol: 0 mg
Sodium: 0 mg
Carbohydrate: 0.8 g
Dietary Fiber: 0.1 g
Sugars: 0.4 g
Starches: 0.2 g
Protein: 0.1 g
Diabetic Exchanges: ½ Fat

Jalapeño-Lime Marinade

This southwestern-style marinade is perfect for grilled shrimp, but it also works well for poultry and pork. Marinate for at least 20 minutes.

1 tablespoon olive oil
¼ cup lime juice
1 clove garlic, minced
1 tablespoon minced jalapeño pepper
Pinch ground cumin
Pinch salt substitute
Dash freshly ground black pepper

Combine all the ingredients and set aside until ready to use. Store, covered and refrigerated, for up to 4 days. Bring to room temperature and whisk before using.

Yield: About ⅓ cup, or 5 1-tablespoon servings

Nutritional Information Per Serving (1 tablespoon):

Calories: 29
Fat: 2.7 g
 Saturated Fat: 0.4 g
 Monounsaturated Fat: 2.0 g
 Polyunsaturated Fat: 0.2 g
Cholesterol: 0 mg
Sodium: 0 mg
Carbohydrate: 1.5 g
Dietary Fiber: 0.1 g
Sugars: 0.3 g
Starches: 0 g
Protein: 0.1 g
Diabetic Exchanges: ½ Fat

Herbed Pepper Rub

Use as a rub on poultry, beef, pork, or lamb. Just rub all over the meat and roast, broil, or grill until done. The mixture can be kept for up to a week, covered and refrigerated.

1 tablespoon coarsely ground black peppercorns
1 tablespoon coarsely ground green peppercorns
1 tablespoon grated Romano cheese
2 teaspoons dried basil
2 teaspoons dried rosemary
2 teaspoons dried thyme
1 teaspoon dried parsley flakes
½ teaspoon garlic powder
¼ teaspoon salt substitute

Combine all the ingredients and stir until well blended.

Yield: 5 1-tablespoon servings

Nutritional Information Per Serving (1 tablespoon):

Calories: 27
Fat: 1.7 g
 Saturated Fat: 1 g
 Monounsaturated Fat: 0.5 g
 Polyunsaturated Fat: 0.1 g
Cholesterol: 6 mg
Sodium: 69 mg
Carbohydrate: 1.4 g
Dietary Fiber: 0.7 g
Sugars: 0.1 g
Starches: 0.1 g
Protein: 2 g
Diabetic Exchanges: ½ Fat

Creole Seasoning Mix

Creole cooking is influenced by a number of cuisines, including French, Italian, German, and Spanish. Jambalaya, perhaps one of the most widely known Creole dishes, is similar to paella, a classic Spanish dish made with rice, vegetables, and meat. This sodium-free Creole seasoning adds Louisiana-style flavor to any number of dishes, including dips, sauces, stews, grilled seafood, and meats, or our own Shrimp Jambalaya (page 122).

1 teaspoon cayenne pepper
1 teaspoon ground black pepper
1 teaspoon ground white pepper
1½ tablespoons paprika
2 teaspoons dried basil
1 tablespoon dried oregano
1¼ teaspoons dried thyme
2 teaspoons salt substitute
1 teaspoon onion powder
1¼ teaspoons garlic powder

Combine all the ingredients and store for up to 6 months in an airtight container.

Yield: 8 1-tablespoon servings

Nutritional Information Per Serving (1 tablespoon):

Calories: 10
Fat: 0.3 g
  Saturated Fat: 0.1 g
  Monounsaturated Fat: 0 g
  Polyunsaturated Fat: 0.2 g
Cholesterol: 0 mg
Sodium: 1 mg
Carbohydrate: 2.2 g
Dietary Fiber: 0.8 g
Sugars: 0 g
Starches: 0 g
Protein: 0.5 g
Diabetic Exchanges: Free

No-Salt Cajun Spice Mix

This mouth-watering mix is perfect for seasoning food before baking, grilling, or roasting and for blackened fish or steak recipes, such as our Cajun Pan-Grilled Catfish (page 115). If you want it to be even spicier, you can increase the amount of cayenne pepper. Unlike most mixes found in stores or used in restaurants, this version isn't loaded with sodium.

¼ teaspoon dried oregano
¼ teaspoon dried thyme
1 teaspoon paprika
1 teaspoon ground cayenne pepper
¼ teaspoon black pepper
⅛ teaspoon ground coriander
1 teaspoon garlic powder
¼ teaspoon salt substitute

Combine all the ingredients and store for up to 6 months in an airtight container.

Yield: 4 ⅛-teaspoon servings

Nutritional Information Per Serving (⅛ teaspoon):

Calories: 6
Fat: 0.2 g
  Saturated Fat: 0 g
  Monounsaturated Fat: 0 g
  Polyunsaturated Fat: 0.1 g
Cholesterol: 0 mg
Sodium: 1 mg
Carbohydrate: 1.3 g
Dietary Fiber: 0.4 g
Sugars: 0 g
Starches: 0 g
Protein: 0.3 g
Diabetic Exchanges: Free

House Italian Dressing

As far as we're concerned, this is the perfect dressing for salads, vegetables, and sandwiches. It also makes a pretty useful marinade. You can adjust the amount of garlic to your liking.

1 cup red wine vinegar
2 tablespoons olive oil
¾ teaspoon dried parsley flakes
¾ teaspoon no-salt Italian seasoning
Pinch ground black pepper
Pinch salt
2 teaspoons finely grated Romano cheese
2 cloves garlic, minced

Mix all the ingredients in a large bowl until well combined. Stir or shake well before using.

Yield: 16 1-tablespoon servings

Nutritional Information Per Serving (1 tablespoon):

Calories: 23
Fat: 2 g
  Saturated Fat: 0.4 g
  Monounsaturated Fat: 1.3 g
  Polyunsaturated Fat: 0.2 g
Cholesterol: 1 mg
Sodium: 14 mg
Carbohydrate: 1.4 g
Dietary Fiber: 0 g
Sugars: 0.4 g
Starches: 0 g
Protein: 0.4 g
Diabetic Exchanges: ½ Fat

Raspberry Vinaigrette

This sweet low-fat salad dressing has very little sodium and is perfect for tossed salads and spinach salads.

3 tablespoons red wine vinegar
1 tablespoon seedless raspberry spreadable fruit
2 teaspoons olive oil
1 teaspoon minced shallot
⅛ teaspoon salt
⅛ teaspoon freshly ground black pepper

In a small bowl, whisk together all the ingredients and refrigerate until ready to use. Whisk again just before use.

Yield: 5 1-tablespoon servings

Nutritional Information Per Serving (1 tablespoon):

Calories: 25
Fat: 1.8 g
  Saturated Fat: 0.2 g
  Monounsaturated Fat: 1.3 g
  Polyunsaturated Fat: 0.2 g
Cholesterol: 0 mg
Sodium: 62 mg
Carbohydrate: 2.5 g
Dietary Fiber: 0.1 g
Sugars: 1.7 g
Starches: 0.4 g
Protein: 0 g
Diabetic Exchanges: ½ Fat

Chunky Blue Cheese Dressing

Low on fat, sugar, carbohydrate, and sodium, this makes a nice choice for salads or to use as a dip. The tofu mimics the blue cheese in flavor and texture, which makes for a chunkier dressing. You can eliminate the tofu and still have a tasty dressing.

2 tablespoons crumbled blue cheese
⅛ to ¼ cup mashed firm low-fat tofu
1 cup light sour cream
3 tablespoons evaporated nonfat milk
1 tablespoon red wine vinegar
1 teaspoon plain low-fat yogurt

Mix the blue cheese and tofu together in a small bowl and set aside for 20 minutes, stirring occasionally.

In a large bowl, whisk together the sour cream, milk, vinegar and yogurt. Stir in the blue cheese and tofu mixture and refrigerate, covered, for at least 3 hours, stirring occasionally. The dressing keeps for up to 4 days in the refrigerator, covered.

Yield: 14 2-tablespoon servings

Nutritional Information Per Serving (2 tablespoons):

Calories: 35
Fat: 2.4 g
 Saturated Fat: 1.4 g
 Monounsaturated Fat: 0.7 g
 Polyunsaturated Fat: 0.1 g
Cholesterol: 7 mg
Sodium: 36 mg
Carbohydrate: 1.9 g
Dietary Fiber: 0 g
Sugars: 0.2 g
Starches: 0 g
Protein: 1.5 g
Diabetic Exchanges: ½ Fat

Honey Mustard Vinaigrette

This light and zesty dressing is perfect for tossed salads and mixed greens or try it drizzled over warm sliced beets, grilled chicken, or steamed asparagus. For an exciting variation, substitute Creole mustard for the Dijon mustard.

2 tablespoons white wine vinegar
2 tablespoons freshly squeezed lemon juice
1 tablespoon Dijon mustard
2 teaspoons honey
Pinch salt
1 tablespoon extra-virgin olive oil

Whisk all the ingredients together in a large, non-metallic mixing bowl until well blended.

Yield: 6 1-tablespoon servings, about ⅓ cup

Nutritional Information Per Serving (1 tablespoon):

Calories: 31
Fat: 2.4 g
 Saturated Fat: 0.3 g
 Monounsaturated Fat: 1.7 g
 Polyunsaturated Fat: 0.2 g
Cholesterol: 0 mg
Sodium: 111 mg
Carbohydrate: 2.7 g
Dietary Fiber: 0 g
Sugars: 2.3 g
Starches: 0.2 g
Protein: 0.3 g
Diabetic Exchanges: ½ Fat

Appendix A:
Health Care Professionals

Certified Diabetes Educator (C.D.E.)

Certified diabetes educators are health professionals who specialize in the treatment of people living with diabetes. C.D.E.'s are certified by the National Certification Board for Diabetes Educators after completing a comprehensive examination and have at least two years of diabetes education experience. A C.D.E. can teach you about a wide range of topics, from meal planning and exercise to diabetic exchanges and blood glucose meters. Try to find a C.D.E. you feel comfortable with who is near where you live.

For more information about certified diabetes educators:

American Association of Diabetes Educators
1-800-TEAMUP4 (1-800-832-6874)
http://www.diabeteseducator.org

National Certification Board for Diabetes Educators
http://www.ncbde.org

Dermatologist

People with diabetes should establish a relationship with a reputable dermatologist who has had experience with diabetes. Sometimes poorly controlled blood glucose levels can cause dry skin and skin irritations. Skin conditions should be taken seriously and addressed promptly before they progress into something more complicated.

For more information about dermatologists:

Journal of the American Academy of Dermatology
http://www.eblue.org

Archives of Dermatology
http://archderm.ama-assn.org

Dietitian

An effective health care team for someone with diabetes should include a dietitian, preferably a registered dietitian (R.D.). A dietitian is a nutrition expert who can tailor a meal plan based on the personal nutritional requirements faced by a person living with diabetes (or anyone else for that matter). Because food is one of the main components of the diabetic lifestyle that requires regulation, a specific diet or eating plan is needed. A registered dietitian has completed academic and work experience requirements set by the Commission on Dietetic Registration. You can use the American Dietetic Association's Nationwide Nutrition Network to find a Registered Dietitian at http://www.eatright.org/find.html

For more information about dietitians:

American Dietetic Association
http://www.eatright.org

Dietitians of Canada
http://www.dietitians.ca

Fitness Specialist

Exercise is an important part of a healthy diabetic lifestyle. A fitness specialist will help you design a personal exercise plan that is safe and effective. Look for a certified fitness specialist who has experience with diabetes, preferably a C.D.E.

For more information about fitness specialists:

American Council on Exercise
http://www.acefitness.org

American Physical Therapy Association
http://www.apta.org

General Doctor/Physician

Choose a doctor who specializes in diabetes and endocrinology, has knowledge of the latest drug therapies, and will work closely with other members of your health care team, including your Registered Dietitian. The American Medical Association offers an online physician search with close to 700,000 listings at http://www.ama-assn.org/aps/amahg.htm

Mental Health Professional

Diabetes can be very stressful. Some people find that consulting a mental health professional, such as a psychologist or psychiatrist, helps them cope with the emotional toll diabetes has on them and their family. Make sure that you choose someone with experience treating patients with diabetes.

For more information about mental health professionals:

The National Register on the Web (Find a Psychologist)
http://www.nationalregister.org

National Institute of Mental Health
http://www.nimh.nih.gov

American Psychiatric Association
http://www.psych.org

American Counseling Association
http://www.counseling.org

Neurologist

A neurologist treats people with nervous system problems. A number of people who have had diabetes for a long time have some type of nerve damage. Find a neurologist who has experience in diabetic neuropathy. Your neurologist should work in conjunction with your general doctor/physician to determine which treatment options best suit your health conditions.

For more information about neurologists:

American Academy of Neurology
http://www.aan.com

Canadian Neuropathy Association
http://www.canadianneuropathyassociation.org

Ophthalmologist or Optometrist

Ophthalmologists and optometrists are specific types of eye doctors. Ophthalmologists are medical doctors with specialized training who are qualified to perform surgery and prescribe drugs. Optometrists diagnose vision problems and eye diseases. They can prescribe eyeglasses and contact lenses, as well as drugs to treat eye disorders, but they cannot perform surgery. Optometrists are not medical doctors, but they are doctors of optometry (O.D.). Look for an eye doctor who specializes in diabetic retinopathy and diabetic eye diseases. It is important to schedule regular examinations to avoid eye-related complications from diabetes.

For more information about ophthalmologists and optometrists:

American Academy of Ophthalmology (find an eye M.D.)
http://www.aao.org

Journal of the American Academy of Ophthalmology
http://www.aaojournal.org

American Optometric Association
http://www.aoanet.org

American Academy of Optometry
http://www.aaopt.org

The Diabetic Retinopathy Foundation
http://www.retinopathy.org

National Eye Institute
http://www.nei.nih.gov

Pharmacist

Pharmacists play a very important part in health care. We suggest that you find a reputable pharmacist with experience in counseling patients with diabetes and diabetes-related health conditions. A personal relationship can be very important, so don't be afraid to introduce yourself and let your pharmacist know a little about your condition(s). Pharmacists are especially helpful in answering questions about new drug therapies, as well as drug interactions and side effects.

For more information about pharmacists:

American Pharmacists Association Foundation
http://www.pharmacyandyou.org

American Pharmaceutical Association (APhA)
http://www.aphanet.org

Podiatrist

A podiatrist is a doctor who specializes in foot-related health care. Look for a podiatrist with experience treating diabetic foot problems. If you ever notice problems with your feet, especially infections or sores, contact your podiatrist immediately and schedule a prompt examination.

For more information about podiatry:

American Podiatric Medical Association
http://www.apma.org

Journal of the American Podiatric Medical Association
http://www.japmaonline.org

Wound Specialist

Look for a health care professional trained in wound care, preferably a certified wound specialist who has experience with diabetics. Having any type of wound can be very serious for a diabetic because of the increased potential that the healing process may be impaired or hindered as a result of your health condition. This specialist must be willing to work closely with your physician in tending to any wounds you may have so they can heal quickly and without infection or complication.

For more information about wound care specialists:

Wound Care Institute Home Page
http://www.woundcare.org

Wound Care Information Network
http://www.medicaledu.com

Wound Care Society
http://www.woundcaresociety.org

Journal of Wound Care
http://www.journalofwoundcare.com

Appendix B: Organizations and Resources

Diabetes and Nutrition

American Diabetes Association
1701 North Beauregard Street
Alexandria, VA 22311
800-342-2383
800-DIABETES
http://www.diabetes.org

American Dietetic Association
National Center for Nutrition and
  Dietetics
120 South Riverside Plaza, Suite
  2000
Chicago, IL 60606
http://www.eatright.org
312-899-0040

American Dietetic Association's
  Nationwide Nutrition Network
http://www.eatright.org/find.html

Center for Nutrition Policy and
  Promotion
U.S. Department of Agriculture
1120 20th Street, NW, North Lobby
Suite 200
Washington, DC 20036
202-418-2312
http://www.usda.gov/cnpp

Children With Diabetes
http://www.childrenwithdiabetes.
  com

Cinnamon Hearts: The Art of
  Winning a Diabetic Lifestyle
http://www.cinnamonhearts.com

Diabetes Forecast
http://www.diabetes.org

Diabetic Gourmet Magazine
http://DiabeticGourmet.com

Diabetic Network
http://DiabeticNetwork.com

Diabetic Newsletter
http://www.DiabeticNewsletter.com

DiabeticShopping.com
http://DiabeticShopping.com

FDA Consumer Magazine
http://www.fda.gov/fdac/

Food and Nutrition Board
500 Fifth Street, NW
Washington, DC 20001
Email: fnb@nas.edu

International Food Information
  Council (IFIC)
1100 Connecticut Avenue, NW
Suite 430
Washington, DC 20036
202-296-6540
http://www.ific.org

Joslin Diabetes Center
Nutrition Services
1 Joslin Place
Boston, MA 02215
617-732-2400
http://www.joslin.harvard.edu

Juvenile Diabetes Foundation
  International
120 Wall Street, 19th Floor
New York, NY 10005
212-785-9500
800-533-2873
http://www.jdf.org

Rick Mendosa's Diabetes Directory
http://www.mendosa.com/diabetes.htm

National Cholesterol Education
  Program and the National Heart,
  Lung, and Blood Institute
P.O. Box 30105
Bethesda, MD 20824
301-251-1222
http://www.nhlbi.nih.gov

National Diabetes Information
  Clearinghouse
1 Information Way
Bethesda, MD 20892
301-654-3327
http://www.niddk.nih.gov/health/
  diabetes/ndic.htm

Nutrition Action
http://www.cspinet.org/nah/

Nutrition, Health, and Food
  Management Division of the
  American Association of Family
  and Consumer Sciences
1555 King Street
Alexandria, VA 22314
703-706-4600
http://www.aafcs.org

ShopForDiabetics.com
http://www.ShopForDiabetics.com

USDA: U.S. Department of
  Agriculture
Food and Nutrition Service
3101 Park Center Drive, Room 926
Alexandria, VA 22302
703-305-2062
http://www.fns.usda.gov/fns

Fitness and Exercise

American Council on Exercise
Consumer Fitness Hot Line
4851 Paramount Drive
San Diego, CA 92133
853-279-8227
800-825-3636

Fifty-Plus Fitness Association
P.O. Box 20230
Stanford, CA 94309
650-323-6160
http://www.50plus.org

President's Council on Physical
  Fitness and Sports
200 Independence Avenue, SW,
  Room 738-H
Washington, DC 20201
202-690-9000

Shape Up America
15757 Crabbs Branch Way
Rockville, MD 20855
301-258-0540
http://www.shapeup.org

Cooking and Food Safety

Daily Diabetic Recipe
http://www.DailyDiabeticRecipe.com

Diabetic Dining
http://www.DiabeticDining.com

Diabetic Newsletter
http://www.DiabeticNewsletter.com

Food and Drug Adminstration (FDA)
Consumer Information Office
5600 Fishers Lane
Rockville, MD 20857
888-463-6332
http://www.fda.gov

FDA's Center for Food Safety and
  Applied Nutrition
800-FDA-4010
http://www.vm.cfsan.fda.gov

FDA's Food Information and
Seafood Hotline
800-332-4010

USDA's Meat and Poultry Hotline
800-535-4555

Related Health Conditions

American Academy of Pediatrics
141 Northwest Point Boulevard
Elk Grove Village, IL 60007
847-434-4000
http://www.aap.org

American Association of Retired
Persons
601 E Street NW
Washington, DC 20049
800-424-3410
http://www.aarp.org

American Dental Association
211 East Chicago Avenue
Chicago, IL 60611
312-440-2500
http://www.ada.org

American Heart Association
7272 Greenville Avenue
Dallas, TX 75231
214-373-6300
800-242-8721
http://www.amhrt.org

American Medical Association
515 North State Street
Chicago, IL 60610
312-464-5000
http://www.ama-assn.org

American Public Health Association
800 I Street, NW
Washington, DC 20001
202-777-2742
http://www.apha.org

Centers for Disease Control and
Prevention
1600 Clifton Road Northeast
Atlanta, GA 30333
404-639-3311
http://www.cdc.gov

Congress for National Health
National Wellness Institute
P.O. Box 827
1300 College Court
Stevens Point, WI 54481
800-243-8694
http://www.nationalwellness.org

Minority Health Resource Center
P.O. Box 37337
Washington, DC 20013
800-444-6472
http://www.omhrc.gov

National Association of Nutrition
and Aging Services
Programs/National Meals on Wheels
1101 Vermont Avenue, NW, Suite
1001
Washington, DC 20005
202-682-6899

National Health Information Center
P.O. Box 1133
Washington, DC 20013
301-565-4167
800-336-4797
http://www.health.gov/nhic

National Institutes of Health
9000 Rockville Pike
Bethesda, MD 20892
301-496-4000
http://www.nih.gov/health

U.S. Department of Health and
Human Services
http://www.healthfinder.gov

References

American Diabetes Association. *American Diabetes Association Complete Guide to Diabetes,* 2nd Edition. Alexandria, VA: American Diabetes Association, 1999.

American Diabetes Association. "Sweeteners." http://www.diabetes.org/main/ health/nutrition/sweeteners/default.jsp (14 January 2003).

Baker, J.L., and B.G. Ostmann. *The Recipe Writer's Handbook Revised and Expanded.* New York: John Wiley & Sons, Inc., 2001.

Hause, A.M., and S.R. Labensky. *On Cooking,* 3rd Edition. Upper Saddle River, NJ: Prentice Hall, 2003.

Schmidt, A. *Chef's Book of Formulas, Yields, and Sizes,* 2nd Edition. New York: John Wiley & Sons, Inc., 1996.

Subak-Sharpe, G.J., and V. Herbet. *Total Nutrition: The Only Guide You'll Ever Need,* New York: St. Martin's Griffin, 1995.

United States Department of Agriculture. "USDA National Nutrient Database for Standard Reference." http://www.nal.usda.gov/fnic/cgi-bin/nut_search. pl (14 January 2003).

United States Department of Agriculture. "Using the Food Guide Pyramid: A Resource for Nutrition Educators." http://www.nal.usda.gov/fnic/Fpyr/ guide.pdf (14 January 2003).

United States Food and Drug Administration. "Food and Meal Planning." 12 May 2002. http://www.fda.gov/diabetes/food.html (14 January 2003).

Warshaw, Hope. "Using the Diabetes Food Pyramid." http://www.diabetes.org/ main/health/nutrition/article031799.jsp (14 January 2003).

Recipe Index

Index